"I have known Russell Feingold persona[...] ever seen him, he has always greeted me with a smile and an open heart. Russell's book uplifts and inspires me with positive (yet authentic) messages and heart-felt enthusiasm. The message of *Heart Wisdom* is the message of Russell Feingold himself: great energy and healing emotions. I love the quotes and the bite-sized, juicy passages. Read and reference *Heart Wisdom* often and experience The Best Day Ever!"

> — *DAVID WOLFE, FOUNDER OF NON-PROFIT THE FRUIT TREE PLANTING FOUNDATION, AUTHOR OF THE SUNFOOD DIET SUCCESS SYSTEM, EATING FOR BEAUTY, SUPERFOODS, NAKED CHOCOLATE, AND AMAZING GRACE*

Russell Feingold is the real deal, and *Heart Wisdom* is a must-read. At a time when the world is hungering for a deeper level of fulfilment, this spiritually profound book has the power to change lives. Tap into your own heart's wisdom and create a life filled with authentic loving and intense joy!

> — *AURORA WINTER, FOUNDER, GRIEF COACH ACADEMY AND AUTHOR OF FROM HEARTBREAK TO HAPPINESS*

Russell Feingold taps into an inner voice that speaks from that quiet space within your heart. *Heart Wisdom* shares a journey of heartfelt determination and is an intrinsically true representation of authentic living. I advise everyone to read, and then to "do" *Heart Wisdom*.

> — *MICHAEL E. GERBER, INTERNATIONAL SPEAKER AND BEST-SELLING AUTHOR OF THE E-MYTH REVISITED.*

"So many people are talking about the heart. Everyone knows love is the answer. Finally someone breaks it down and shows you how to access the Great Treasure within, and finally release the burdens of debilitating pain and suffering! Thank you Russell for this outstanding work to set us all free – Truly brilliant!"

> — *JILL LUBLIN. INTERNATIONAL SPEAKER AND BESTSELLING AUTHOR, GUERRILLA PUBLICITY, NETWORKING MAGIC AND GET NOTICED GET REFERRALS*

"Russell Feingold is an extraordinary healer with a remarkable ability to both correctly diagnose and heal energy blocks."

— *ARIELLE FORD, BESTSELLING AUTHOR OF THE SOULMATE SECRET*

"Russell gently takes you by the hand to unwind the stress, tension, and fear that has prevented you from having the life you truly desire. Working with Russell Feingold will permanently excavate the hurt and suffering, replace your pain with peace, regain your sense of trust and motivation, and reboot your ability to freely give and receive love again."

— *L.A. WEEKLY'S "BEST OF L.A."*

"Russell Feingold is one of those rare jewels that you discover in this wonderful life. His ability to help others tap into their God-given gifts and live in their own true power is phenomenal. Having worked with both Deepak Chopra and Wayne Dyer, I can honestly say that Russell is in their league."

— *MICHELE BLOOD, AUTHOR AND TV SHOW HOST OF MPOWERTV.COM*

"I have had the good fortune of working with Russell on numerous occasions over the past 10 years, as a personal coaching client and a participant in many of his programs. I am constantly amazed at his profound ability to get to the core of all issues with such wonderful ease, love and grace. Simply amazing!"

— *DAWN PILJEK, FOUNDING PARTNER OF VITAL LIFE WORLD, DELRAY BEACH, FL*

"Russell Feingold may serve as a model for other Inspirational Leaders and Life Coaches. He has an uncanny ability to discern between "The Story" and the underlying Truth of what is really happening in people's lives. Russell brings a perfect blend of compassion, fun, and unrelenting realness to his clients and students. He leaves you with only one option… to choose to change your life."

— *JOSHUA MACK, LMT, HEALER & TEACHER, FOUNDER OF HANDS ON WELLNESS*

"Russell Feingold is an extremely gifted coach. His ability to get right to the point in those areas needing attention is amazing. His holistic approach to the challenges I am facing goes deeper than ordinary conventional coaching, making lasting changes inevitable! I recommend anyone who really desires long term change to contact Russell immediately, you owe it to yourself!"

— *NEVILLE HANCHETT, REAL ESTATE INVESTOR*

HEART WISDOM

Your Transformational Guide To Joyful Living And Loving

RUSSELL FEINGOLD

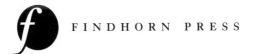

FINDHORN PRESS

© Russell Feingold, 2010

The right of Russell Feingold to be
identified as the author of this work has been asserted by him
in accordance with the Copyright, Designs and Patents Act 1998.

Published in 2010 by Findhorn Press, Scotland

ISBN 978-1-84409-533-9

Edited by Gemini Adams, Sandra Sedgbeer, Nicky Leach
Cover design by Dan Yeager
Interior design by Damian Keenan
Printed and bound in the USA

1 2 3 4 5 6 7 8 9 17 16 15 14 13 12 11 10

Published by
Findhorn Press
117-121 High Street,
Forres IV36 1AB,
Scotland, UK

t +44 (0)1309 690582
f +44 (0)131 777 2711
e info@findhornpress.com
www.findhornpress.com

Contents

Disclaimer

This book is not intended to be a diagnosis, prescription, or cure for any specific kind of medical, psychological, emotional or spiritual condition. The author, the publisher and their employees, and agents are not liable for any damages arising from, or in connection with the use of this book. Each person has unique needs and this book cannot take these individual differences into account. For specific treatment, prevention, cure or general health consult a licensed, qualified physician, therapist or other competent professional or practitioner.

From the Author

I stand in awe and with deep respect for the miracle that is life, and for the courage it takes to walk your authentic path. I am humbled by your willingness to do the work that is necessary to unravel your conditioned reality and liberate the love of your immaculate heart. May your journey be graceful as you delve inward to excavate the hidden jewel that is your deepest truth— the miraculous, living intelligence that is the heart of life itself. The road can be challenging at times, though I have found nothing more rewarding than the cultivation of Heart Wisdom. If someone had told me what lay within "I never would have believed 'em..."

MY GREATEST WISH FOR YOU:
That you discover the astonishing light of your own being
and drink of the infinite love within your heart!

I have heard people say that in order to create something big, your "why" must be really BIG. Well, I tell you that the time came in the creation process of this book, when the "why" became irrelevant. It didn't matter what the why was anymore. I just knew I had to do it... Something deep within me, from the depths of my soul grabbed hold and compelled me to *get what was inside me out. Heart Wisdom* had taken on a life of its own. It was relentless and wouldn't give up. It claimed my life and wouldn't let go until what needed to be said was said. And that was that. And that was enough!

During the process, it was like I was living to get this book out into the world. At the same time, I was amazed at how much solace I received each time I read a portion of the book. It was my saving grace during some rather crazy times in my life and in the world. I would read, and then feel that everything was going to be okay—that I am okay . . .

And it was.

And I am.

Acknowledgments

How can words express the gratitude of a dream being fulfilled? By thanking the people who made it possible! Each person listed here has touched my heart and enriched my life in extraordinary ways. Their love and care for me are woven through these pages and the pages of my life. Their contributions will have an impact among those whose hearts heal and lives become transformed through the experience of Heart Wisdom.

Thank you

Geoff Feingold: my brother from the same mother. I am honored, and proud and grateful to have you as my brother. Should all siblings be so lucky.

Brother Rawsheed: All hail the Justice League, and God bless our eternal brotherhood— deep love. You are profoundly Heart Wise!

Kute Blackson: My brother of the heart, thank you for your precious friendship, guidance and support in helping me stay true to the path. You are a mountain of Heart Wisdom—'nuff said!

Jason Corburn: My oldest and dearest friend. What a long, strange trip it's been. You are a profound blessing in my life and your friendship is gold!

Kim Delaney: You were *Heart Wisdom's* first midwife. Thank you for helping to make this possible. (Special thanks to Kevin Delaney because you just rock!).

Aurora Winter: My coach and trailblazer of the heart. Bless your impassioned vision for the healing of grieving souls. May the Grief Coach Academy soar to immaculate heights of success and service! Thank you for your enthusiasm, support and inspiration.

Howard Lipp and ena vie (and Sweetums): Ah, yep! What to say? Millions of miles, infinite worlds—still alive to tell about it, and to share more laughs, and many more magical moments.

Gemini Adams: *Heart Wisdom's* second midwife. Goddess bless your patience, and vision, and steadfast belief in me and this work. Thank you beyond measure!

Jill Lublin: Dear friend, maestro strategist and PR maven, bless your beautiful spirit and generous heart! Thank you for your relentless encouragement in always believing in me, seeing my greatness and holding me up in my most brilliant light. With you, there is no such thing as "can't" or "fail" or "give up." There is only the great news of "Truth that must be shared!"

Lisa Schneiderman: The love we shared has served my heart's blossoming in ways I could never explain. Bless you, and thank you!

Special thanks to all of my clients for your trust and faith in me, and for your invaluable "field work!" This book has come to life from your courage and willingness to dive deep inwards to heal your magnificent hearts, and to restore peace to your lives and the world.

Brian Hilliard: Thank you for being love, and always bringing it!

Rene Jenkins: You are magic and one of my greatest musical inspirations.

Janay: Bless you, sweet angel,

Jill Mangino: Thank you Boo Boo, for your love, support and humor—you make me laugh!

Damiani Sekoulidis: You are simply a treasure.

Shimshai: For your infinite blessings of musical medicine.

Sita, Ayasmina and Nicola: For the precious and invaluable work you do—you have blessed me beyond measure.

Thierry Bogliolo of Findhorn Press for believing in the vision of *Heart Wisdom*.

And to Mother Aya: All hail the Queen… *¡Ay, caramba!*

Also, thanks to Dan Yeager for cover design, Kris Clark, Judah Schiller, Anthony Bottoli, Jude and Eti Kodama, Jeff Happy Bear, Richard MB, Joshua Mack, Bruce Suggs, Gloria and Gwen Jones, Debbie and Arielle Ford, Michael Mamas, Oscar Miro Quesada, Nina Murphy, again Mom and Dad, Deb Feingold, Erik Rabasca, Carlos Booy, Dr. John Burchard, Brandon Fox, Deepak Ramapriyan, Mike G., Duke Hillinger, Stephanie Lana, Gogo, Christo Pellani, Deborah and Matthew Mitchell, Ryan Wookie Mitchel, Laurie Grant, Shelly, Freddy and Stacey Strauss, David Wolfe, Keval Ohri, Melanie Benson Strick, Jacqueline Hadden, Govindas, Sunny Solwind, Miranda Rondeau, Niki Breit, Miki Knowles, Dawn and Sasa Piljek, Mateo Daniels, Max Simon, Ella Lauser, Kim Riccelli, Scott Vineberg, Yogi Hendlin, Fabiano, Deb and Yuri, and the whole Circosonic family—I love you all!

And last, but certainly not least, my angel Sandie—my final editor, my agent, my friend, my savior! You have cared as much about this book as I do, and sometimes it felt like even more! You have believed in me, the power of the heart and the message of *Heart Wisdom* so far above and beyond. Bless your radiant British heart and your colossal integrity. You have a heart of gold and you are truly Heart Wise! And as true as this statement ever was, "This would not have happened without you!" Few are the words to express the depth of my gratitude. You know how I feel .

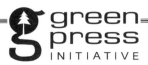
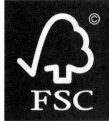

Dedication

I dedicate this book to my parents, Helene and Robert Feingold, two people in my life who never gave up on me. We have not always agreed, and, as with all parent-child relationships, we have endured our share of challenges. But when all is said and done, you have always been there for me, and have always loved and supported me. Mom and Dad, I love you both so dearly, and am blessed to have you as my parents. Thank you for believing in me, relentlessly caring about me and helping my heart's wisdom to blossom.

This book is also dedicated to my dear friend and spiritual sister, Teresa. Teresa suffered a spinal cord injury about four years ago in a snowboarding accident. Since that time she has been devoted to her healing and committed to a full recovery. She has made great progress and is well on her way!

Teresa—very few people can relate to what you go through on a daily basis. You demonstrate more courage, strength and heart in one day than many people will in their entire lifetime. You are a precious gift and a living inspiration to this world! You have given me so much through your strength and courage and perseverance of heart, that I have chosen to donate a percentage of the proceeds of *Heart Wisdom* to honor you, support your healing and celebrate your immaculate heart. Thank you, Teresa, for being you, and for being a living example of Heart Wisdom. I love you dearly. Shine on, sweet Teresa! My heart will always walk with you.

To find out more about Theresa and her miraculous healing journey, visit her Web site at: *www.peruvianproject.org*

Prologue

Enlightenment is not a place in the geographical sense. Yet countless flights have been booked, guidebooks written and passports renewed in quest of it. My own pursuit of this bliss has taken me to India, Nepal, Peru, Los Angeles, Florida, Las Vegas and Vancouver, to name but a few places. I have also taken many courses and programs, read countless books and absorbed the content from hundreds of tapes, CD's and DVD's.

Every step in the journey took me closer, but it was one trip, my farthest trip—to Pune, India—that revealed to me that the source of enlightenment—the liberation, fulfillment, peace and bliss of that which I now recognize as Heart Wisdom—was much closer to me than I had imagined. It was then that I fully comprehended what Heart Wisdom really meant. Prior to this trip, I had thought that wisdom, or enlightenment, was "out there." I had no idea I'd been carrying it with me each time I packed my bags, or that I could access this incredible guidance without sitting atop a mountain in the Himalayas or praying on a special mat in some far-flung temple.

I had decided to take an intensive course in craniosacral balancing at an ashram in India on the recommendation of one of my teachers. Craniosacral balancing is a form of bodywork in which the practitioner connects to the wavelike rhythm of your cerebrospinal fluid flowing in and out of the dural membrane. The dural membrane envelops the brain and spinal cord, thus supporting your body's natural ability to heal and be healthy. The first time I connected with the craniosacral rhythm, bells went off for me. This rhythm and the ability to work with it to promote, support and honor the body's innate wisdom to heal itself seemed to be the mother of all healing arts to me.

The course ran for eight weeks, with seven hours of practical work every day,

Sundays included! When it was over, I had the opportunity to extend my time into a 10-day intensive doing multiple-hands craniosacral work. By this time, I had been at the ashram for about two and a half months and was deeply embedded in the life there. Feeling very open to everything, I signed up for a three-day meditation course, which used a process, called "Who is in?" For those three days, we were isolated from everyone else at the ashram. The idea was to take away distractions in order to provide the conditions for our attention to move out of our heads, inward. With this uninterrupted inward focus we would be able to pierce the veil of our illusions and move away from who we thought we were into who we really are in our truest self. Well, this was the idea anyway!

To support our spiritual journey during the "Who is in?" course, we were given special food. It was bland and designed to be nourishing but not savored. We were instructed to avoid eye contact and conversation except when we performed the "Who is in?" dyadic exercise (meaning between two people), which we did about eight times a day.

Every morning, we'd wake up at 5 a.m., move to the center of the room and sit down in front of a partner. I mean, literally. One moment you are asleep, and then the next, your eyes are open and within minutes you are sitting in front of someone staring into their eyes! This was the only time you were permitted to look at someone the entire day. Then, one person would ask the other person one simple question: "Who is in?"

For five minutes you then relate your experience, which includes anything that is going on for you at that moment. It might be "I'm sick of being here," or "I miss my family," or "The food sucks." It might be a tenderness or soreness in your body, or the feeling of the floor underneath you, or a sense of joy, pleasure, even bliss. Whatever happens across the screen of your experience is the exact answer to the question "Who is in?" After five minutes, the gong sounds, you say thank you and switch. This time you ask, "Who is in?" and the other person talks for five minutes.

You go back and forth like this for twenty minutes, and then you bow and move on to the next activity (i.e., group meditation, a meal, sleep). There is no more eye contact or talking until your next "Who is in?" exercise. These sessions are not meant to be a two-way conversation: the purpose is for each person to ask the question not connect. You are to remain open as an empty vessel. Your attention is to be 100 percent inwardly focused.

I had already gone through several courses at this center, and had been regularly meditating for years at this point, so it was relatively easy for me to get out of my mind chatter and focus inward. As a result, the first day flowed beautifully and blissfully for me. I was conscious of my body feeling comfortable; my mind felt relaxed and filled with loving and peaceful thoughts.

However, on the second day the exercise got a little tougher. While seemingly subtle and simple, the practice was working me a little deeper than I thought. Things began coming up. This was my stuff—baggage that I'd been carrying around. It was intense, and my mind started flailing. The "stuff" grated on me, and I felt anxious and agitated. My mind began making up stories, twisting the feelings I was experiencing as my ego fired in reaction. I felt out of control, my mind racing, everything was rubbing, grinding, grating against me. The friction increased.

It was as though these thick, tough ropes were constantly being rubbed against my head, faster and faster, until they began to be chewed up and shredded. Finally, the very last thread on the very last rope snapped, and SWOOSH: the hot air balloon was flying free—the puppet became free from the puppeteer. Something gave way deep within me and completely released itself. My mind unhooked, my heart opened, the incessant chatter abruptly ceased. The Hindus call it "Samadhi," an essential state of freedom in which the mind is perfectly still, perfectly free.

After that practice I went outside and stood with the trees. I moved more freely than ever before. I was laughing and giggling like a small child. And I realized that I was part of an exquisite flow that ran through me, and all around me, yet there was no "me." I stood among the trees feeling the fresh air and released my laughter to the breeze. I had been shaken free of my mind chatter—free from the insanity of caring about what others might think, of my old stories and fear-induced excuses.

As my mind quieted and all of the veils of illusion dissolved, all that was left was "my" heart and the wisdom therein. The realization struck me: I had been given the profound gift of being shown the path to my own liberation. It was a gift that had always been there waiting for me.

This breakthrough completely changed my experience of life. I was fulfilled in that instant. It felt like I had just popped open. Even my vision was clearer. Colors, words, details—everything was exquisitely crisp and vibrant. I understood now that there was a much deeper reality, another way to live—another place to be and to come from.

I had accessed my heart and become fully immersed in the wisdom of the Universe that flows through it. For the first time in my life, I knew what it meant to be in tune with my true self. It was one of the most wondrous moments of my life; yet, what happened to me in Pune had very little to do with my geographic location. Although India is a kind of Mecca for enlightenment seekers, I could just have easily been in Idaho.

Did my experience bring me enlightenment? Maybe yes, maybe no. What I am clear about is that it was a moment of tapping in to the flow of the Universe, with all its innate wisdom. I was able to experience what it is like to live without kinks in the hose, free of all the mental and emotional restrictions that we create for ourselves through stress, drama and dilemma. I experienced what I call *Heart Wisdom*: the freedom to follow your bliss, the ability to recognize and connect with your authentic self and to receive guidance that is appropriate for your soul. That was when I realized that liberation from pain, doubt, misery and suffering is—and always has been—just a heartbeat away.

HEART FACT

"The average heart beats 110,000 times a day, 40 million times a year, 3.5 billion times in a lifetime."

When you make that deep heart connection and access your own heart wisdom your life changes dramatically. You may realize that you think differently and feel differently than you used to, and you move through life's experiences with a new sense of ease and grace. If we all were able to move from head-centered thinking to living our lives from this wondrous heart wisdom we could become co-creators of a much more healthy and harmonious world. The only thing that stands in our way is the belief that "something" outside us prevents us from doing so.

From the Great Abyss to Bliss

We all struggle with the insanity and enormity of the Infinite. When we witness the incredible beauty of the sun slipping into the ocean, or feel the breeze dancing across a meadow, or when we see the serenity and joy between loving couples, we are provided with a glimpse of this awe-inspiring bliss. But these experiences often cause us to retreat into our tiny safe spaces—our patterns, habits, ruts and addictions. We feel secure in the knowledge that we can't possibly have or deserve such greatness, even though we know, on some level, that happiness is possible, right here, right now.

But we don't trust happiness. Instead we revert to the fallacy that we must wait until something has been achieved to be happy. We tell ourselves the "if only" lie—"If only I had the perfect relationship, a bigger paycheck, a little more time in the day, (fill in the blank _____), *then* I would be truly happy. The truth is, happiness doesn't exist in the past or the future; it can only exist in the now. Anything else is just a *thought* of happiness. How many times have you passed up what might have been a wonderful opportunity to experience happiness in the now with a subtle act of self-sabotage born of this fear?

Breakthrough experiences like the one I had in Pune have shown me that we don't have to wait for that immaculate day to come when all will be bliss. Bliss is not in the tomorrow of our lives! Bliss is here. We all have the ability to create the life we truly love, right here, right now… and to go on creating it—moment to moment, day to day. For many years, I sought to understand a feeling I had that something "wasn't quite right," to shine light on it, and find the path to a greater sense of fulfillment. My own journey through this abyss helped me to discover the power of Heart Wisdom, and it changed my life.

Having made this discovery and experienced the incredible and profound benefits that come from living from the heart, it has been my immense joy to share my insights and lessons with many people—clients, readers, family and friends. I have served as a guide, supporting them as they released their old "baggage," including the subconscious conditioned patterns and limiting beliefs that had influenced their minds and steered their lives. I have offered assistance as they sought a place where they could "lose their mind" and come to their senses. I have shown them ways to stop intellectualizing and get out of their heads, so they could drop into a deeper sensory and experiential intelligence. In so doing, they have been liberated from struggle, opening the door to infinite possibilities and bringing a clarity of mind that empowered them to manifest their heart's greatest desires.

Where are you coming from?

When people ask each other, "Where are you coming from?" they really mean, What brought you to this point? In one sense, "Where you are coming from?" is your past, everything that has made you who you are. While you can't change your past, the truth is, when you know who you really are, you *can* change where you are coming from at any given moment. Most of us spend our whole lives not knowing our true selves because we are coming from our heads. But if you've already felt that not working for you, then it's time to tap into your heart's wisdom and access your best life… right now.

When we live from our heads we rationalize life rather than experience it. We derive our truth from a mental/intellectual place, rather than a sensory, feeling experience. We rely on what we know, rather than what we feel. But that is illogical. It's like trying to comprehend the intensity of the sun from reading about it in a book, as if the word "sun" has anything to do with the reality at all. That is absurd. As a dear friend of mine says, "You can't get wet from the word 'water.'" Yet that is how most people live their lives—by hearsay, at best—and in so doing have become inured to the actual experience of life. They have forgotten that precious jewel within their own hearts, and feel disconnected from its joy; for within the heart, there is a profound wisdom that not only exists but is readily accessible.

Once you realize that this wisdom exists—that there is another way to live and that, in fact, operating from our Heart Wisdom provides us with an infinite number of wonderful ways to live in this abundant Universe—there is no going back. The only option is to continually push away the boundaries that have held you back—the boundaries of what you thought was You. Now, go to your edge and open your heart to what's just beyond that. Each time you reach your edge, look down into the mouth of the dragon, then dive in, something (you) breaks free a little (sometimes a lot). Something great is stirred, shifted and transformed. What remains is a sense of awe, a strange kind of awkward yet graceful gratitude.

From that point on, the answer to the question, "Where are you coming from?" is forever changed. Your "polarity" reverses. You go from living almost entirely with your attention in your mind—with a river of energy in your mind and just a few currents of awareness in your heart—to living with your attention firmly in your heart with only the necessary currents of awareness in your mind.

Of course you still use your mind, but when you are living from your heart the relationship between heart and mind shifts. Now, the mind serves the heart—encourages its greatest expression, its greatest loving—and with this new relationship the whole Universe becomes accessible to you. When you live from your heart, you allow your authentic self to guide you in all your choices, rather than being guided by some societal construct, pressure or standard. But what is amazing is how effortlessly every aspect of your life—relationships, career, family, finances, fitness, attitude—begins to fall in line with your dreams.

Where I am coming from?

During the past fifteen years I have worked with thousands of people, and in the process have developed a methodology to quickly and easily guide you inward to the deeper intelligence of your heart's wisdom. This is actually very simple, yet it is something we were never taught! This process, which had its genesis in the culmination of my experience in Pune, and which has been refined over the years into nine simple yet profoundly life-transforming keys, will help you release your old "baggage," including the subconscious programming and limiting beliefs that have been directing your mind and your life since earliest childhood. This process, which I refer to as the Heart Wisdom Process, will lead you unerringly to the wisdom that is rightfully yours. It is this gift that I now wish to share with you.

Throughout this book, we will explore the path to your heart's liberation. As we journey through this transformation together, I will introduce you to these nine keys and show you how to use them to reach your Heart Wisdom consistently to effect rapid and lasting change. Connecting with your Heart Wisdom will help you clear the contractive patterning that has held you back from stepping into your full potential and feeling the full force of your authentic power. It starts with YOU—the deepest and perhaps even buried YOU that is directly connected through the heart to all that is the Universe. Connecting with that deep, essential YOU is the gateway to the greater truth that will set you free. This is a practice that will change your life.

These nine keys, when used together, provide the spark that will set your whole world on fire. You will open to a ravaging love—a veritable volcano of vitality, passion and joy! In these pages, you will learn exactly what you need to do to plug into the power of your heart's wisdom and access the fantastic life that is available for you. The concepts and exercises you find here will guide you in letting go of all the stress-creating habitual patterns that have been holding you back from creating the life you want and feeling truly fulfilled and happy.

In this book you will learn all about Heart Wisdom and the infinite power it has to fuel and nourish your life. You will also learn about the most common modes of contraction—those things that block the flow of heart wisdom into your life. You will cultivate a practice that will enable you to tap into your heart wisdom and continuously deepen, refresh and stay open to that connection. This practice will also help you reconnect in a heartbeat if a contraction develops.

In the final section, you will learn how to integrate Heart Wisdom into every aspect of your life. You will also learn how to stay open to this connection in any circumstance or situation. When you use this knowledge and the practical tools in this book, you will not only ensure access and openness to your Heart's Wisdom but also learn how to stay open to this connection in even the most challenging circumstances.

As you become adept at using the Heart Wisdom Process, and gain the knowledge and understanding of your own Heart Wisdom, you will intuitively and easily respond to situations that used to confound you or cause you grief. Life will become sweeter and more peaceful regardless of what may be going on around you. And you will enjoy an incredible sense of liberation, because you will know reality from your heart rather than from your head

The Stakes

There is much beauty, joy and opportunity in the world, but there is also very real suffering and pain. Until we are willing to acknowledge this truth, recognize it within ourselves and acknowledge our own contribution to it, we will continue to contribute to the pain and suffering, thereby perpetuating a way of being that is unnatural and destructive on a personal and planetary level.

The end result of living from our heads over many generations is that we have lost any conscious, tangible understanding of our abiding connection to nature and to each other. Today, we experience our global connection mainly through trade, war, new technologies, and so on, but we are connected on a much more intimate level as well. This is not some trite, idealistic, "New Age-y" concept; it is a deep truth that not only forms the foundation of every spiritual and religious tradition but is substantiated by extensive scientific research.

To understand this, we only have to realize that the air we breathe is circulated through all of life—we actually share one breath. The air also is a carrier of more subtle components of energy that fill the space as well as make up all things. In that sense, all of life is connected by and as energy. It is who we are and what we share.

When we allow our hearts to atrophy, this awareness and sensitivity deteriorates; we literally lose touch with the essential truth of our interconnectedness. As a result, most of us continue to live almost completely from our minds and disconnected from our hearts. We create a world of scarcity and fear—right here in the middle of an abundant Universe.

Many of us recognize that something is "wrong." Perhaps that's why you've picked up this book. In the popular science fiction film *The Matrix,* Morpheus explains this situation to Neo:

> *"Let me tell you why you're here.*
> *You're here because you know something.*
> *What you know, you can't explain; but you feel it.*
> *You've felt it your entire life.*
> *That there's something wrong with the world.*
> *You don't know what it is,*
> *but it's there, like a splinter in your mind,*
> *driving you mad".*
> — *MORPHEUS (THE MATRIX)*

Until we wake up and acknowledge our own connection and personal contribution to the greater whole, we will continue to perpetuate suffering.

As a side note, you will find that I make a significant number of references to the film *The Matrix.* The first time I saw it, I walked out of the theatre and sat down on some steps; I was so altered and utterly transformed, I was virtually unable to move for about 3 hours! There are some experiences in life that are such epiphenous moments that they shake us out of our reality and bring us back home to the truth. This was indeed the case for me in seeing, or should I say experiencing the paradigm shattering cinematic phenom known as *The Matrix*!

Today, the world is experiencing its own modern-day matrix-like Renaissance of sorts. You can see it reflected across the spectrum of life, whether it be the economic, business, social, political, environmental or ecological arenas. The heat has been turned way up, and change—big change—is at hand. The question is: What are you doing to prepare for it? How are you contributing to it?

I offer this book as a bridge between the world that is just now departing and the one that we are just now entering, to empower and support you in awakening to the immaculate, transformational force that not only lives within you but *is* you. Acknowledging this force, and integrating it into your daily life, will best equip you to deal with whatever may arise in your life.

HEART WISDOM WARM-UP

Preparing to Read from the Heart

I suggest you read through this exercise a couple of times to become familiar with it before you embark on it in earnest. Alternatively, you can go to the Heart Wisdom Web site (*www.heartwisdom.com*) and download the free MP3 recording I have made to guide you step by step through this exercise.

I invite you to begin your journey by reading this book differently, with a different awareness—an awareness that comes from your heart. Traditional reading is done from the head. If you read from the head, you will more or less stay engaged in the head. This book is designed to bring you into your heart. Now is the perfect time to start practicing reading from the heart:

- Take a deep breath.

- Bring your attention to your breath.

- Follow your breath in through your nose and down into your pelvis. Inflate your abdomen like a big Buddha belly and continue to let the breath inflate up into your heart.

- Hold your breath and allow your attention now to rest in your heart.

- Let your heart soften. Then let the rest of your body relax into your heart.

- When you're ready, exhale your breath while maintaining your attention in your heart.

- With your attention in your heart, continue to breathe and begin to read.

This takes practice, and just this practice alone will transform your life. If you find yourself drifting into your head or your mind gets distracted, re-engage the breath, inflate into your heart and relax your attention into your heart. You have this entire book to practice.

CHAPTER ONE

Freeing Your Mind of Clutter

The mind is a terrible Master
but a wonderful Servant.

— VIVEKANANDA

If you are reading this book, it is undoubtedly because you want to create change in your life; yet to do this, you need to be clear about both what it is that you desire to change, as well as what you wish to invite into its place. As the internationally recognized personal development trainer T. Harv Eker explains, "Most people don't get what they want because they don't know what they want." Awareness is the first step to transformation.

It is important to recognize that if you don't know what you do want, you will, for the most part, keep getting what you don't want. More often than not, this comes about because we are living from our heads, not our hearts. And the mind cannot possibly know what it is that the soul desires without accessing the heart.

The Chattering Mind

The mind's primary role is to organize, manage and deal with information—information that already exists and needs to be processed. Thus, by its nature, the mind is rooted in the past. However, the mind also exists as pure potential. When healthy and connected to the heart and its wisdom, the mind is available for us to use as a vehicle, to be programmed for our benefit—to analyze the data presented to us in our everyday situations. When the mind is "unhealthy," or disconnected from the heart and its wisdom, it *thinks* it is the center of attention, and instead of being able to effectively use our mind for our own benefit, our mind uses us.

One of my favorite bumper stickers reads: "Don't believe everything you think." Many people function as if whatever reveals itself in the canvas of their mind is actually real and, therefore, necessitates action! They don't create the time or space to pause for thought, meditate or allow for real clarity to arrive from their "inner voice." The chattering mind smooshes together with messages from the overpowering emotions, and before you know it you're doing something that just isn't quite right. If we don't create space from all the mental noise, we can't discern what is real, empowering or warrants our attention over what should be ignored. We react, rather than respond.

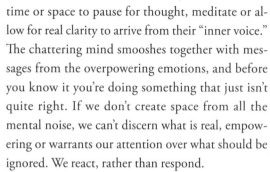

HEART FACT

"The heart has its own nervous system consisting of over 40,000 neurons. Neuroscientists call this "the brain in the heart."

Unfortunately, Western culture has evolved in a way that has conditioned us to keep our attention in our heads. Our entire schooling system is designed to educate us into our minds, placing primary importance on convergent thinking, on getting the right answer or being right. Sadly, with so much value placed on being right, that is what we strive for. We have become a head-driven society, and we have developed patterns in our lives that reflect a "heady" existence.

One of the unfortunate byproducts of this way of thinking is that most of us experience incessant mind chatter and have difficulty slowing the mind down. For many people, this is what they consider to be their normal state. For others, the mind goes into overdrive when they are nervous, or stressed out. The thoughts, ideas, debates and conversations just keep chasing themselves round and round, like a dog chasing its own tail.

The mind's tendency is to fixate, to attach itself to certain issues or worries. It *thinks* its job is to keep us safe. It does this by preoccupying you with what is known and familiar—things that have already occurred. This way you won't make scary plans or take risks for the future. That's why your mind so often talks you out of creating big changes in your life. The voice you hear inside your head—as opposed to your "inner voice"—might tell you it's too hard, it's never going to work, it's too late. It will provide you with a thousand reasons, just so you will maintain the status quo.

The mind thinks it is the "center of attention." It thinks it is it, the whole kit-and-kaboodle! This is the trap that keeps you stuck in your own head. It is the essence of egoism and arrogance—the very antithesis of love, compassion and understanding. When you come from this place, your relationship with life unfolds accordingly. As you perceive people and experiences from this mind-centered place, you attract experiences and people that reflect the same ego-centered, safety-orientated, limited outlook.

Because of our desire to feel safe, we let the mind run the show. But this is actually not safe at all. It prevents us from having growth and vitality. It stunts our expansion by keeping us locked in the past, locked into old and unproductive patterns of thinking and reacting. For example, when you feel fear, if your mind is conditioned or patterned to shut down or run away, you will always react in this way, never getting present to work with the fear.

When we live from our heads like this, we get stuck. If we let the mind run the show, rather than our hearts, we will never achieve our dreams or reach the fulfillment we so desperately desire, which is not surprising when you consider that the human mind, left to its own devices, is unreliable at best.

When we live in our minds, we are like a tornado. The brain thinks in circles, so we get caught up in a kind of spinning pattern that our actions follow. We do more and more, yet somehow never get to a place where we feel fulfilled. We create more and more restrictions in our lives as we take on more projects and responsibilities to fill our calendars, and yet nothing ever feels complete. We think, "Someday, when I've made enough money, or done enough work, or whatever it is for you, *then* I will be (fill in the blank: happy/content/relaxed) _____.

We keep ourselves so busy, yet the more we do the more we feel we need to do, and that "someday" slips farther and farther away. The truth is that the more we do, the less we do authentically. The modus operandi for so many of us is "do, do, do"so that you can "have, have, have," and then you can "be." This way of functioning will lead you to be having a lot of doo doo! You'll probably get burnt out and you won't ever achieve peace, pleasure or satisfaction. Instead you'll end up living in a place of insanity (or at the very least quiet desperation), one that cannot possibly lead to the liberation and fulfillment you so deeply desire.

Another problem with "head-centered" living is that whatever we are holding onto in our minds will prevent us from being fully present and open to our Heart Wisdom. Information that hasn't been processed that

31

is left floating in the mind draws our attention and drains our energy. As David Allen, author of *Getting Things Done*, so succinctly puts it: "That which you hold in your mind takes up 'psychic RAM.'" Really, the mind is seeking to know itself. It does this by seeking your attention. But the mind can never know itself from its own perspective; there must be space for this to occur. And for this to happen, you must move into a place of greater observation or witnessing.

In order to free your mind, you must move beyond it. To see its truth, you must let it go; otherwise, it's like trying to see your own face without looking in the mirror. The mind may be a fantastic processing and creative center, but it's a horrible storage facility. What is not efficiently processed will eat up your energy, constantly pulling at you on a conscious or unconscious level, depending on where the event, story or concept is "filed" in your mind. Allen's main focus is encapsulated in the Eastern martial arts concept—Mind Like Water—used to teach students to maintain a state of mental fluidity to keeps things off their mind, so their minds are open and their energy remains free.

> **HEART FACT**
>
> "The electrical impulses generated by the heart are 40 to 60 times stronger than those generated in the brain. The heart has the strongest electrical impulses in the body."

In essence, the mind is an organizing intelligence. It is not the source itself, though most people function as if it is. Their attention is directed from the mind, as opposed to the heart. And they create their reality from a mental space and then wonder why they are unfulfilled. Fulfillment is qualitative. The mind is not a qualitative experience; it is a function. If you come from the head, you will create a mental reality that can never satisfy your heart.

When you drop out of your mind, and move into your heart, the mind becomes reoriented to a more powerful place. A different relationship unfolds in which the mind becomes a powerful source for analysis and implementation, where it isn't in control and doesn't need to be in control. A greater intelligence is running the show and it comes through as Heart Wisdom.

Living this way has immeasurable benefit, not just for the body, but for our entire being. A deep letting go ensues, and the body opens to a profoundly vital place of deep peace and relaxation. When the energy of life merges with the physical body, instant transformation can happen. This is the gateway to true fulfillment, a place where you can experience enlightenment, living authentically, joyfully and lovingly.

Avoiding Authenticity

So what is holding us back from moving out of our heads and into the infinite wisdom of our hearts? More often than not it is fear—fear of authenticity, fear of being seen, fear of failure. It is a fear that is caused by our limiting beliefs, negative self-talk and overactive emotions, which choke the bliss out of our hearts and restrict our ability to freely and fully express who we really are.

It starts when our minds convince us that we don't know how something will work out (so you had better not try it), or "talk" us into believing that we can't possibly ever be all that we desire to be. Alternatively, something happens, a situation or circumstance that instantly evokes a negative emotional reaction. Fear, grief, worry and anger—any of those powerful, paralyzing emotions set your heart pounding, blocking you and stopping you from doing what you know in your heart you really want to do.

And so, instead of living "your bliss" and creating an authentic life, you continue chasing your tail, letting your chatty mind and reactive emotions put fear into your heart, canceling and drowning out the wisdom that is so desperately trying to show you "the way." Consequently, you end up living a frantic or restricted life, making reactionary choices based on the limitations of your mind, beliefs and emotions.

Have you ever noticed those people who seem to be over the top, forcing it? Well, the truth is they are over the top, and they are forcing it. They certainly aren't living from their Heart Wisdom. Rather, these are the kinds of people whose reality is artificially driven by the thoughts in their heads and their overactive emotions. They are so far removed from their hearts that they fill whatever the perceived need is in the moment through compensation. Such people may appear "pumped up," but their bodies have, in fact, contracted as opposed to having opened from within.

Pumping yourself up in this way comes from a powerful inner need to prove something or to perform in some way. The mind interjects itself into a situation and says, "Okay. We aren't good enough for this. We have to prove something now. Let's get it together." So the energy gets pulled from within the organs, namely the adrenals, with a resulting "adrenaline" rush. This has the desired effect of making the person "feel" great, but only temporarily. Eventually, this inefficient strategy for living will lead to burnout, misery and a lack of fulfillment.

Living in this kind of frenetic do-ing way only distracts you from your Heart Wisdom and from being in touch with your true self and the gifts you have to offer the world. You start to "do" for the sake of doing, instead of doing in order to share your gifts with the world and find your bliss. If you are constantly doing, accomplishing more and more, it's hard to know whether you are authentically inspired and passionate or just charged up on your own adrenaline.

Even when we seek to change our lives, we tend to use this frantic approach. We fit even more into our lives so we can initiate the desired change: books, programs, seminars, diets, exercise routines, and then we have to work more so we can afford to pay for it all. Mercifully, the point of this book is *not* to get you to work really hard or clutter your life anymore in order to bring about change. This isn't about getting something or "finding" yourself. It's about helping you realize the truth. You're right there already. Actually, you are right here already! You have just forgotten.

When you are grounded, connected to your "inner voice" and have a balance between the mind and the heart, your energy is channeled and distributed efficiently and precisely. You won't burn out from proving something to the world. Instead, you'll gain clarity, connection with others and a deep sense of satisfaction, because you are able to live authentically and follow the path that suits your soul.

When we get addicted to distracting ourselves in the ways I have just described, we create massive blockages to our ability to connect with our Heart Wisdom. We simply stop opening. The result of this is a terrible sense of being unfulfilled, disappointed, incomplete and let down.

This was certainly my experience before I had that moment of realization in Pune. Prior to my trip, I had been creating my life from a head-centered place focused on looking to external sources for my satisfaction, outside in, if you will. My ability to freely express myself was severely impaired. I spent many frustrating hours caught up in the endless chattering loop of my mind, as it told me to do this rather than that, creating illusory reasons as to why I shouldn't be doing the things that my soul seemed to crave.

But I needn't have traveled thousands of miles to discover that I could end the pain and suffering that this way of life had caused. And neither do you. You can release the restrictions that prevent you from living in your heart, following your authentic self from wherever you are right now.

Checking In

Before we go any farther, I'd like you to check in with yourself and see if you are still reading from the heart or has your attention wandered back to your head? If you find you are "stuck" in your head, just take a few minutes to shift your attention back to your heart by doing the breathing exercise found at the end of the prologue.

When your energy and mind are both clear, when your heart is open and you are connected to the wisdom within, you allow a much deeper intelligence to function in your life. It's like the difference between driving a car that's operating on two cylinders and one that's firing on all eight! You can literally feel the difference, can't you?

If you are not connected to your heart, you have no way of navigating this world—no way to discover who you are, where you come from, and what you are doing here; your purpose will always elude you. Conversely, when you live from your heart and not your head, you are constantly plugged into the Source. You are in the flow, connected with the essence of who you truly are and totally at one with your infinite self. There's nothing to fear and nothing to force, because everything you want or need flows effortlessly toward you, like iron filings to a magnet.

According to California's Institute of Heart Math, which is investigating the relationship between the heart and the earth's magnetic field, evidence suggests that when we are present and heart-centered, every system in our body entrains to heart coherence. The beauty of it is that we already have a cord connecting us to our heart's wisdom; we just need to know how to plug it into the right place to create a connection with all of life and its possibilities.

The nine keys outlined in this book are purposefully designed to take you on a journey from your head into your heart, where you will experience your true and infinite self. By connecting to your Heart Wisdom in this way, you get to reach the core of your being and access the power that will enable you to create the life you truly desire. From here, you can discover what it is that your soul—your authentic self—*truly* wants. Only in this way can you ever be fulfilled.

The Nine Keys

In the remainder of this book you will learn exactly how to do this by using the nine keys of the Heart Wisdom Process. I developed these key specifically to access the joy, love and abundance that is rightfully yours. At the end of each chapter, you will find practical exercises and a deeper understanding of one or more of the nine keys to accessing your Heart Wisdom.

The nine keys to accessing Heart Wisdom are:

1. Learn how to free your mind of clutter

2. Become conscious and aware of how you seek and find fulfillment

3. Use your breath to turn your attention inward

4. Identify the contractions within your body

5. Learn how to release blocked emotions

6. Find forgiveness

7. Connect with love you thought you had lost

8. Integrate your Heart Wisdom in your body and in your life

9. Live your Heart Wisdom and experience unity with others and the Universe.

The nine keys outlined in this book are designed to help you dissolve all the obstacles and restrictions that have been standing in your way. Once you start playing with them, you'll be surprised at how quickly you'll be able to calm your inner chaos, master your own mind and become fully present. When you open to the divine guidance of your Heart Wisdom, you cannot help but see things differently.

When you change the way you look at things, the things you look at change. You will begin developing the inner practice that will free you from the limitations of stress, anxiety and confusion and catapult you from "heart-breakdown" to "heartbreak-through." In this way, you will reconnect with the clarity, love and joy that already lie within you.

But before you can do this, you will first need to understand how you are presently seeking and finding fulfillment. This is important. Not only because it will help you know yourself a little better, but also because it will help you understand why and how the rest of the Heart Wisdom practices and exercises in this book will benefit you. We are all seeking fulfillment. It is this search for "the one thing" that will fill the hole within us that can be our greatest blessing or our worst curse.

Completing the following exercise will reveal a lot about how you habitually seek and find fulfillment now. As you move through the exercises in this book, you will be able to turn your attention and focus towards finding fulfillment in new and better ways. Now is the time to step up to the plate, examine your patterns with a compassionate yet realistic eye and prepare to find true fulfillment through your own Heart Wisdom.

HEART WISDOM KEY NUMBER ONE

Freeing Your Mind of Clutter

Many of us struggle to find out what our gifts are. The technique below is designed to help you center your awareness and open yourself up, so that you connect with the heart wisdom that will guide you to this knowing. As you connect with your authentic self, your unique path will become clear. But first you need to create "space" to open the channel to access your heart wisdom.

Most people try to get to know their mind by being immersed in it, overthinking, overanalyzing and never having a clear picture of what's going on in there. It's like trying to read a book with your nose in the binder. You've got to give it some space. As a thought comes into your head, it's important not to focus on the thought itself, but how you deal with it. Realize that it's your response to the thought that matters, not the thought itself. Sometimes it is helpful to explore where the thoughts are coming from. Sometimes it's not. You have to be present with your thoughts as they come up.

When working with my clients, I tend to use the question, "What comes to mind?" as opposed to "What are you thinking?" The reason for this is that the former generates an authentic heart-centered response, one where the listener can maintain awareness, while the latter causes the listener to travel right back to the merry-go-round of the restrictive chattering mind.

You may complete this exercise on your own, or you can go to the Heart Wisdom Web site (*www.heartwisdom.com*) and download the free MP3 recording I have made to guide you step by step through this exercise.

So let's start by turning your attention inward toward your mind. Be aware of your thoughts (what comes to mind) as you relax into the infinite space of your consciousness, but don't get caught up in them. Be a curious spectator. See each thought as a cloud in the sky. Where there are not thoughts there is only blue sky. Your mind in essence is a clear, infinite blue sky and the thoughts are intermittent visitors.

In the beginning it may seem quite overcast, with some interspersed patches of blue because your mind will likely be clouded with thoughts. That's okay. Start by being aware of the spaces *between* those thoughts. Look for the patches of blue, so to speak, and relax into them, if even just for a moment. Each time you are aware of a thought coming into your field of perception, let it pass.

You don't have to try to do anything with the thoughts that are floating in your mind. Just let each thought float by, blessing them as they pass. By simply allowing them to exist and letting them move on instead of focusing on how you can't seem to stop them from happening, you avoid trapping them in your mind. Before long you'll be experiencing clearer and clearer "mental skies" because you will be freeing your mind of cluttering thoughts.

CHAPTER TWO

Seeking and Finding Fulfillment

*All things, material and spiritual, originate from one source and are related as
if they were one family. The past, present, and future are all contained in the
life force. The universe emerged and developed from one source, and we evolved
through the optimal process of unification and harmonization.*

— MORIHEI UESHIBA

Whether we are conscious of it or not, we all live our lives seeking greater
fulfillment. Some call it enlightenment, bliss, inner peace or content-
ment. The problem is that labels can get in our way. Rather than get caught up
on what it is called, just go with the flow, have the experience and call it whatever you want later. The underlying desire isn't to find a name, but rather to find
something that literally fills us up—fills our time, fills our minds, our hearts,
our bellies—so that we can finally feel *good.*

The sad truth is that most people, when willing to be totally honest, admit
they are unfulfilled, frustrated and wish their lives were different. In part this
is because we tend to look for fulfillment in our outer world, in other people,
sex, our careers, food, alcohol, drugs, even seminars and self-help programs. Yet
if we truly understood the nature of fulfillment, we would know that we have
been looking in all the wrong places. Typically these "dangerous" temptations
come in three guises: God, sex and money.

The Seeking

God, sex and money are the primary driving forces for many people in the
world. We get conflicting messages from all directions in the media, advertis-
ing and popular culture, motivating us to take certain actions, often on the
false promise that fulfillment is right around the corner. Yet, if you consider the

definition of fulfillment: "Fulfillment is being healthy on all levels, experiencing an exquisite balance of functionality and harmony with your life. It comes from being at one with who you are and in total alignment with what you are choosing to create in the moment."

More simplistically, fulfillment means being fully filled with who you really are, not who you *think* you are. When we look to money as a means of fulfillment, we are reaching outside ourselves for that which can only be provided internally. A life geared toward accumulating more and more money does not create the conditions for "being healthy on all levels." On the contrary, it creates the conditions for both continual disappointment, as well as a continual need for more and more. This is not to say that to want money is bad—not at all. Rather, it's the unhealthy fixation on money, and the more-more-more mentality that often results from it that is the killer.

Looking to sex for fulfillment has a similar outcome, as well. At its best, sex is pleasurable, exciting, healing and even transcendent! Unfortunately, many people don't experience this wonderful exchange in this way. For them, sex is about power, "getting off" or having their ego satisfied. Yet, unlike money, sex can be an incredible vehicle to access your inner world, to connect with your true self and to open the heart to its wisdom. This can certainly be the case for those who practice the ancient art of pure Tantra, as it takes them on the ultimate journey in living and loving from the heart instead of the head.

Looking to any god for fulfillment is perhaps the most complicated and unsatisfactory method of achieving authenticity. Like Heart Wisdom, God exists inside us. When we live at our highest level—when we are tapped in and connected, our actions aligned with God—we can then experience life in a joyful and loving way; fulfilled and content we can then live from an authentic place. Yet many religious belief systems present the idea that God is external, a judgmental force in our lives, rather than a source for love, creativity and guidance.

This has us searching outside ourselves again—being fearful of others' judgments of our behaviors and decisions. Being dependent on any external authority for approval makes it extremely difficult to listen to your "inner voice" or connect to your Heart Wisdom. This is because looking to an outside authority for validation fools you into believing that the source of wisdom must lie outside you, when in fact your heart *is* the only source of truth. It cannot be any other way, because the heart knows *only* truth.

Know Thyself

Problems occur when we start judging ourselves in relation to how much money or sex we have or how religious or spiritual we are. These comparisons become the determining factor in how we value ourselves or compare ourselves with others. Fulfillment is really about being healthy on all levels; it comes from experiencing an exquisite balance of functionality and harmony in life and from being in total alignment, relaxed in who you truly are and focused on what you are choosing to create in the moment.

Fulfillment involves aligning "where you are coming from" with what you are doing. It comes from aligning the head with the soul, which can only be achieved through the wisdom of the heart. The challenge is that few of us know how to access this wisdom. How could we, when few of us think of the heart as anything other than an organ that pumps the blood and oxygen around the body, or something that gets us into romantic and emotional trouble!

The heart is so much more than this: it is the gateway to the soul, the opening to a deeper wisdom, the place where we can literally feel what is "right or wrong" for us. By understanding how to access your Heart Wisdom and practicing this, you can find the fulfillment you desire and create the life you truly want to live.

Since you are reading this book it is fair to assume that the earlier quote by Keanu Reeve's character Neo in *The Matrix* that "there's something wrong with the world… " strikes a chord within you. The question then becomes not *if* this is true, but *how deeply* do you understand it? Too much focus on external distractions and not enough focus on your own heart's wisdom may be robbing you of the joy and bliss that is your birthright.

Do you keep asking, "Who am I?"

If you often find yourself feeling lost, lonely and wondering why nothing ever seems to be enough, then it's likely that you are stuck in your head and disconnected from the wisdom of your heart. The other symptoms of this may manifest as a general sense of malaise or low-grade depression, or feeling like you are spinning on the hamster wheel of life, never getting to the juicy bits that you so desperately desire. It's as if your life is playing out like an old out-of-focus black-and-white silent movie, yet you could swear that somewhere in your psyche, there's a deep knowing that sometime in the past, you were operating in dazzling full-color 3D.

*Do you have unsatisfactory relationships
with yourself and others?*

Do you find that you are stuck in obligatory or disempowering relationships with friends, family or colleagues? Are you doing things you think you "should" rather than because you can't wait to do them? Do you feel that you aren't being heard and have lost interest in listening to others? If the answer to any of these questions is Yes, then you are disconnected from the wisdom of your heart. In more intimate relationships with lovers or spouses the symptoms will appear as a lack of intimacy, passion and excitement, and the sense that you just aren't getting your needs met.

HEART FACT

The source of the heart-beat is not in the brain but in the heart. When a heart is transplanted it cannot be reconnected to the brain, and yet it beats beautifully on its own.

*Do you want to connect with
a new passion
and sense of purpose?*

Does your life seem flat? Do you look at others with a tinge of green envy and wonder, "How come their life is so damn cool?" Have you always sensed that you were here to do "something" important, but never had the time or know-how to figure out what that might be? If any of this sounds familiar, it's a sign that you're disconnected from your heart's wisdom and living more in your head. Passion and purpose come from the heart, not from the head. You cannot rationalize your way into your heart to discover your purpose, let alone ignite your passion!

Do you want to make clear choices
that will truly serve you?

If you find that decision-making is "traumatic" for you, or that you always make the wrong decisions and end up in situations that don't serve who you really are, then it's most likely because you are making decisions only with your head, without engaging your heart and its greater wisdom. By learning how to access the heart, you will discover an unerringly accurate way to weigh up the pros and cons of your life choices. Supported by a greater intelligence, you will find the path to effortless decisions that continuously serve your soul and your life.

Do you wish to become awake, alive and thrive,
rather than struggle to survive?

If you've been struggling through life, and are exhausted by battling along in survival mode, then you are suffering from the "Lone Ranger syndrome": you are thinking and believing that you must go it alone. You are disconnected from the greater intelligence that will aid and support your soul in its journey, ignite your passion, and keep you awake, alive and vibrant in the flow of life. The only way to this place is through Heart Wisdom—a journey you will surely want to take.

Do you want to remove physical stress
and spiritual suffering?

If you've been trained to live from your head and have been fighting your way through the game of life, then you will notice a number of side effects that may have begun to emerge: Tiredness, depression, laziness, a lack of motivation, even more severe signs that might have manifested as physical illness or disease. Spiritually, you may also be experiencing some form of pain. You may not notice it during the busyness of the day to day, but at night while lying alone in bed, especially on a Sunday night, or even while relaxing on a retreat, suddenly those feelings of emptiness and a lack of fulfillment surface. Somewhere inside you sense the suffering of your soul. It's sadness that you didn't make the choices that would have guided it toward its purpose, or made the contribution you came here to make. Is that how you want to spend the remainder of your life? Or would you prefer to discover how you can experience a joyful and loving life? Now!

Unused Potential

Now imagine, for a moment, that you are a high-powered computer. Although you are available and powered with infinite potential, you spend much of your day stuck in sleep mode, waiting for something to do, something to compute, so that you can fulfill the purpose you were created for. This is how so many of us live our lives. We have the potential but it remains unused because our systems are clogged up with all the old programs, data and mind viruses that we don't even recall downloading and installing. We might make an effort to upgrade our software, spruce up our operating system and explore a few new programs just to see what we're capable of achieving, but either the operating system doesn't support all them, or there are system conflicts caused between new programs and their older versions. Better play it safe—stick with what we know. Maybe someday someone else will come along and recognize our potential and make everything work for us. Only someday rarely comes. Time passes. Frustration sets in. Our equipment begins to falter, we get damage to our hard-drive and the screen begins to fade. How does this show up in our lives?

- We want to move forward but subconscious baggage keeps sabotaging our efforts to change;
- Limiting thoughts, beliefs and belief systems prevent us from trusting ourselves and others, which severely limits our ability to give and receive;
- Unresolved emotional traumas keep tripping us up;
- Painful past memories keep replaying in our head, the anxiety they cause then gets projected onto the future, magnifying our fears of taking risks;
- Chronic frustration, anxiety and fear not only lead to depression but also impact our immune system, making us susceptible to disease and illness;

- Unresolved emotions and tension cause blockages in the body, which in turn can lead to headaches, migraines, physical pain and illness.

This can be described collectively as our "conditioned reality," more commonly known as our "stuff." It's this "stuff" that holds us back from accessing our Heart Wisdom and finding lasting fulfillment. Unfortunately, the degree to which we are unaware of the influence of these patterns and programs on our thoughts, beliefs, attitudes, responses and behaviors is the degree to which we are unable to experience this deeper fulfillment.

Over the course of our lives—especially from birth through four years of age—we are incredibly impressionable. During those first four years, when we learned how to live and survive through the relationship and experiences of our parents, we were imprinted with their programs and belief systems about life, relationships and the world. How they communicated, dealt with situations, processed their own emotions, understood themselves and the world around them, related to others, and how they functioned or expressed love within re-lationships are all programs that were imprinted into our subconscious minds (our operating system).

As we grew up and began to live our own life, these parental programs have continued to run in the background, covertly influencing our perceptions, silently directing our inner thoughts and behavioral patterns, and ultimately shaping our world. And so long as we keep on doing what we have been condi-tioned to do, we will keep on getting the results that we have always got.

The Practice

This is how we have progressed as we have gone from one generation to another, passing these negative programs learned from our parents, grandparents and an-cestors down our lineage. In the process, we have forgotten that we are all one. And what is remarkable to notice is that what occurs within us is reflected right back to us in the outside world. For example, if you are experiencing chaos in your outer world, this is a sure sign that there is some chaos that is left unmanaged in your inner world. Thus, if we want peace, we must find it within ourselves. If we want a more abundant world, first we must access the abundance within.

Unfortunately, most of us continue to live almost completely from our conditioned minds, and as a result, together we create a world of scarcity and fear—right here in the middle of an endlessly abundant and astonishingly generous Universe. Thankfully, more and more of us are now acknowledging that there is something wrong with this picture. Deep down we know that isn't why we are here or where we are really coming from. The feeling that something is wrong eats away at us.

If there is one thing we all have in common and know deep in our spiritual bones, it's our need for purpose, connection, and meaning. Humanity is waking up to the fact that the materialist value system that has dominated our society simply doesn't work for our greatest benefit—collectively or individually. When we are caught up in the endless pursuit of getting—whether it's material possessions or relationships with people—we are completely dependent on something outside ourselves to feel valuable and happy.

The desire and quest for this false happiness can even lead us to disregard the effects of our actions on our fellow humans. In one moment it may seem that a certain item of clothing, like a new shirt, will make us finally feel like we belong or that we've made it. Yet because we are so focused on the temporary fulfillment of our own self-gratification, we may not even consider or care about the conditions behind the production of this shirt.

Perhaps the shirt was made by poorly paid Indian workers who are stripped of their rights and forced to endure horrifying treatment (the kind that would make you cringe if only you knew the truth). Maybe the fibers for the cloth were grown with harsh pesticides and then exposed to processing chemicals that subsequently seep into the land and water affecting the natural balance of the ecosystem, and perhaps the workers then breathe in the chemicals.

Despite this chain of destruction, we still buy the shirt. And still happiness and fulfillment eludes us. So we move on to the next object, the next desire that we must fulfill in order to reach that elusive place of happiness. In a lifetime of chasing fulfillment, just imagine the wreckage one person can leave in their wake.

To realign our individual value system and that of our communities, countries and ultimately, the world, we must regain a balance with nature. We must develop a practice that connects us to our inner world so we can access our Heart Wisdom and let it flow through us. When we do that, we naturally make the choices and actions that support health. If we can learn to access this place, everything else will fall into order.

When we allow ourselves to be fulfilled from within, we will then make our business, lifestyle and purchasing decisions from a place of completeness instead of lack. As a result, our need to be filled up with material things, achievements, relationships or sex starts to dissolve. When we live from a place of fulfillment, we create an entirely new and more satisfying experience and also, not coincidentally, make the world a better place.

HEART WISDOM KEY NUMBER TWO

Become Conscious and Aware
of How You Seek Fulfillment

This exercise provides you with a wonderful opportunity to grow in consciousness and awareness—to become. You must be prepared to be as honest as you can in order to become aware of the unfulfilled needs that are motivating your choices and shaping and evolving your experiences and your life. Consider this exercise an experiment and don't skip it, because it is a key to understanding where you are coming from so that you can shift more easily into your Heart Wisdom. At the end of this book, we will return to this exercise and use what you write in your journal today as a yardstick to measure how much you have grown and changed through the Heart Wisdom practice.

1. Take a blank sheet of paper or your journal and make a list of all the major items that you have either bought or desired in the past six months in the belief that they would make you happier on some level. Include all the things you thought you wanted that you acquired, as well as all the things that you don't feel you have, but you want. This includes material possessions as well as other desires such as promotion at work, professional recognition, success in business, new friends, a committed relationship, and so on. It doesn't matter what form the desire takes—if it's something that you want but don't yet feel you have write it down. (Think hard about this and don't let yourself off the hook.)

2. Now write down all the things that you would love to be able to have or buy in the next six months.

3. Next, write down next to each item how you think your life
    will be different when you have the item, person or achieve-
    ment you wrote down in step two. What will it give you? How
    will you feel? And what is the overall impact you think it will
    have on your life?

4. Alongside each of the items you have already listed explain why
    you think that particular item will make you happy. What is it
    going to give you that you don't have now? What is that thing
    going to add to your life, your personality or your reputation,
    and so on?

5. Once you have completed your list put it away in a safe place
    because we will be using later.

CHAPTER THREE

When Inner and Outer Worlds Collide: Turning the Focus Inward

I only went out for a walk and finally
concluded to stay out till sundown,
for going out, I found, was really going in.

—*JOHN MUIR, ENVIRONMENTALIST*

We are all aware that we have an inner world, one that can be both silent and loud, yet always private. Unfortunately, it is a place many of us rarely visit. This is the world of thoughts, emotions and feelings—of our energy, consciousness and relationship to other living beings. We know it exists because we hear our inner voice speaking words or instructions that we may never dare to repeat or act upon in the outer world. Sometimes we access this inner world through our dreams—where we experience the innate intelligence of this world as it reveals details and meanings that can help us better understand and interpret the happenings of our outer world experience.

Other times, when our life seems hectic or out of control, we crave the silence that can be found within our own core, the peace that lies beneath the madness of the mind, a space of serenity that strangely remains hard to find. Yet this inner world is our direct line into the wisdom of the heart, to the greater intelligence of the Universe that can guide and direct us on the path that will serve our soul. The question, therefore, is how do we reach this inner world in order to access our Heart Wisdom?

The Natural Way

In both my own experience and from the work I do with my clients, I have found that too many of us have almost completely severed our ties from our inner and our outer nature: the trees, the mountains, the earth. Sitting with our inner world "stuff," our deepest emotions, desires, traumas, and even joys, is not a practice that is encouraged in Western society. As a result, exploring our inner world can be disorienting—more like traveling in a far-away country than returning to a familiar homestead.

Being in and connecting to nature allows us to connect to our true essence, as well as our sacred relationship with the earth and all living things. Our connection to nature is ancient. It is a well-lit pathway to the Universe and to our inner world. This is why visionaries like Muir, Christ, Lao Tzu, and Thoreau immersed themselves in nature in order to connect with their deepest truths. And it's why even a short hike into the forest can bring us back to ourselves, clearing the mind, opening the heart, to leave us feeling nourished and refreshed.

Unfortunately, in our contemporary society, it is more common for nature to be a distant notion that we experience only rarely and with some degree of discomfort and vulnerability. One of the most startling ways that this disconnection shows up in our outer world is through the current climate crisis. In neglecting our inner world, we have forgotten and literally lost touch with the intimate relationship and ancient connection that we once had with Mother Nature and the earth.

HEART FACT
Your heart cells are the first cells that form when you are a fetus in your mother's womb.

This connection between our relationship with our inner world, nature and the ongoing humanitarian and environmental crisis is not as abstract as it may seem. Consider that our inner turmoil leads us to create a life of seeking that is not in alignment with our true values or purpose because we are not guided by the wisdom of our hearts. We want to be fulfilled—truly, madly, deeply—yet we are trained by marketers and advertisers to look for that fulfillment in products and services, not in our inner world or in nature. We are constantly looking for that *something* to fill us up and make us feel better.

We cannot make choices that will serve us from this place of nonalignment, yet every choice we make has an impact on the world we live in. When we pause to look closely and follow the rabbit hole of these decisions, we can see the undeniable evidence of the role we play in creating a globalized society that is structured on a good portion of the world's population staying poor, one that continually violates their human rights, and one that does not honor and care for its precious natural resources—the earth, water and air that we all need to survive.

But many of us are more intimately connected to our material goods than our Heart Wisdom, and to our minds rather than nature. This is a problem, a big problem. If, just for a moment, we can dare to turn off the iPod, pop the bubble and look directly at the deep, dark shadows of our society and ourselves, then we can begin to grow personally and as a species.

When we are truly connected to our inner world and, thus, to the earth, we cannot help but act in ways that preserve and nourish this deepest part of ourselves and the collective. The truth is our world has turned outside in because we are turned inside out! The average person in the United States spends 90 percent of each day indoors. We have so completely severed ourselves from the Great Outdoors, that to say that nature is part of our inner world may seem confusing. But spending time in nature is one of the easiest ways to connect to the inner world and access our inner nature so that we can tap in to our Heart Wisdom.

Outer-world landscapes of human-made meanings and materials have eclipsed our inner world and taken over what we now feel is essentially "us." I would be willing to bet that most people's primary concern isn't nature, or how to connect with it, but how their life fits into society. No doubt, their considerations center around what defines them as human, what makes them worthy, of value, what announces their identity and status to others and what is expected of them because of those signals. When you operate from this premise, your authentic self and all that is natural remains hidden from your daily reality. This is why we so often feel lost, stuck and as if we're spinning our wheels, going around and around in ever-decreasing circles.

The Outer World

The outer world is the scene you create or the one that is happening around you. The outer world is often a reflection of how you treat your inner world. If you aren't connecting and conscious of your inner self, it can show up in your bank account (are your payments up to date?) In your bedroom (does it look like a bomb exploded?) In your home (is it a chaotic mess that drains your energy or a cleanly organized retreat that nurtures and rejuvenates your spirit?) And your car (does it look more like a trash receptacle or a respected chariot to take you where you need to go to offer your gifts to the world?) The outer world is made up of your material possessions, your interactions, day-to-day situations and the landscapes you've created as the setting for your day-to-day life and how you interact with all of these external elements.

In this outside-in world many of us have created, we often feel more connected to those material things and situations or identities in our outer world than we do to our inner world and our essential selves. The Apple iPod is a classic example. People treat this material object as an intimate part or extension of themselves, staying continuously hooked up to the device in order to have a constant soundtrack to their lives.

Instead of tuning into their own inner music—the vibrations of the earth, the Universe, and the life that plays beautifully inside each of us—such people tune into 60 GB of outer-world music. Instead of sharing their own inner music with others, they share outer world playlists as a way of interacting, impressing and forming relationships with others. Song and genre choices stand in for true selves. When used consciously, music can be a powerful aide for opening us to our inner selves, but the mindless drone of the iPod can drown out our inner world messages and keep us stuck in our outside-in worlds. The continuous musical stream and the ever-present ear-bud can actually obstruct the path to our own inner world by distracting us with external noise.

So how does all this inattention and distraction, this disconnection and isolation show up in our lives? Let's take a look at the collective outer world. Consider the extent of poverty in the world; approximately 850 million people are malnourished and nearly seven million children die every year from malnutrition. It's astonishing to think that in this world of plenty, one-fifth of the world's population, or 1.2 billion people, are living in abject poverty, meaning their situation is desperate and life threatening. Even in our own backyards, there are homeless people, neglected elders, abused children, animals and adults and our world economy is in a disastrous state. Our "house" is certainly not as well cared for as it could be.

So what does this mess have to do with you and how you're living your life? You aren't taking food from impoverished people's mouths or money from their hands. Yet the truth is that the suffering of the world is a direct reflection of the turmoil and lack of connection in each of our inner worlds. When our inner worlds are disconnected and in shambles it shows up in our own outer world.

For example, when we struggle to fill the spiritual hole by buying stuff, we can end up with a cluttered and uncomfortable environment that doesn't make us feel good at all. When each of us fails to take care of our inner world "stuff," the outer world stuff gets worse, it gets magnified and the collective effect is the eternal suffering and tragedy that we witness on the nightly news. We have to recognize that our inner world is one interwoven, multidimensional consciousness that we share with the Universe, which means that how we treat our inner world is literally how we treat ourselves—and our inner worlds show up in our economics and our environment.

Global Warming is no misnomer, and scientist have already attributed melting glaciers, increased sea levels, more severe hurricanes and other storms and greater intensity of droughts to this cause. The heated debates between scientists and officials from prestigious universities to the United Nations have ended; the discussion has now moved on to assessing what the damage is and how it can be prevented. What is not being considered, though, is how our individual behavior toward ourselves affects the natural environment. Global Warming is a symptom of the pain we cause the earth, the culmination of centuries of abuse to "self" and Mother Earth.

It is not surprising that the indigenous peoples, who often serve as a voice for the suffering earth and the need to care for it, have for centuries been abused or destroyed. But the hard truth—or the "Inconvenient Truth," as Al Gore calls it—is that the storms and other natural disasters that have, and will, continue to cause so much misery are the actions of an intelligent organism taking care of itself, acting out of self-preservation. Going back to the science fiction film *The Matrix* again, we find a great illustration of the reason for this as Agent Smith tries "to break" Morpheus:

I'd like to share a revelation that I've had during my time here. It came to me when I tried to classify your species and I realized that you're not actually mammals. Every mammal on this planet instinctively develops a natural equilibrium with the surrounding environment, but you humans do not. You move to an area and you multiply and multiply until every natural resource is consumed and the only way you can survive is to spread to another area. There is another organism on this planet that follows the same pattern. Do you know what it is? A virus. Human beings are a disease, a cancer of this planet. You're a plague...

But there is a solution. When we are connected to our inner worlds, we do achieve equilibrium with our surroundings because we feel our connection to the earth as much as to our own flesh and blood. We feel the pain of the earth, and because of that, we make conscious decisions, aware that the pain is unbearable and that we need to put a stop to it. When we feel this connection, we realize our contribution to the world at large. Remaining unconscious perpetuates a way of being that is devastatingly unsustainable. The longer we ignore our inner worlds, the more pain we create for the earth and the worse the economic and environmental crisis will get.

Turned Inside Out

Once a month I used to lead a night hike through Topanga Canyon, a gorgeous green space in the Santa Monica Mountains just northwest of Los Angeles. The aim of this group activity was to help everyone connect with nature, harmonize with his or her heart and get away from the preoccupations of the mind so they could heal their outside-in orientation.

Only one person showed up to the first hike I led in this particular series. Having expected at least 10 people, I was a little disappointed but recognized it as a great opportunity for me to surrender my expectations and trust the unfolding of this experience. I reminded myself that the perfect people always show up at the perfect moment and that Divine perfection is always at play.

Susie, the sole participant who showed up, was pretty flustered when she arrived. Obviously in a hurry, and stressed out about everything going on in her outer world—her job, her car, the traffic—she started organizing the "stuff" she was planning to take with her, pulling things from the trunk of her car. Suddenly a gigantic flashlight appeared. When I asked "What's that for?" Susie explained that she felt safer with it because we were going out into nature in the dark. I thought about the situation from her point of view. She was going out into the wilderness in the dark accompanied by a man she didn't know! It quickly became clear that the flashlight wasn't only intended to light her way, it was also a potential weapon for whatever or whoever might threaten her along the way—me included! Understanding Susie's position, I let her bring the flashlight, after I had made it clear that she could use it only if absolutely necessary. She agreed. So we set out in the dark. The dank coastal fog pressed against us, and although we were outside, I felt claustrophobic. At times we could see no farther than a few feet in front of us. During the course of the walk, we would stop periodically to bring our awareness to the nature around us.

After spending all day in the big city that is Los Angeles, it was actually jarring to be in such a quiet space where we could hear every individual sound, including some rather eerie animal ones. I'll admit that although this hike was my idea, my companion wasn't the only one who felt a little nervous! We were totally unprotected from the wild. There could have been snakes or mountain lions anywhere. But what might seem crazy is that we weren't looking to be protected from nature; we were trying to open ourselves up even more to it.

Susie shared how disconnected from nature and how out of her comfort zone she felt. As we were walking, those feelings intensified for her. At one point she seemed to collapse in on herself. I asked, "What's happening for you right now?" She expressed that she was experiencing fear. So I supported her through an "unraveling" process that began with a few questions: What do you think the fear is about? What's preventing you from being totally at peace right now? What would have to happen for you to feel okay? Susie had to delve deep inside of herself to find those answers. We took our time and created the space for her to feel safe and to sift through all of the emotions that were coming up for her.

First she accessed her inner world and found the courage to trace the fear. Memories of a traumatic event in her childhood soon started to surface. Susie had been traveling in a car with her friends' parents, and they had driven off the road and got stuck out in the middle of nowhere. Because the adults she was traveling with were clearly scared to death of being alone in the wilderness, they were unable to create a sense of safety and comfort to allay Susie's fears. For young children, adults represent total authority. They're older, wiser and so much more knowledgeable than children are; ergo, if an adult is scared, there must *really* be something to be scared about. Unsurprisingly, the adults' fear became magnified and imprinted in Susie's psyche. The trauma she experienced that night effectively ended Susie's relationship with nature.

As we ventured out into the dark wilderness that night, all those long-suppressed feelings and fears came back to "haunt" her. And, brave girl that she was, she turned herself inside out, allowing the unconscious "stuff" to unwind and rise up to the surface so that she could finally release it and set herself free. That night, Susie liberated herself. She found her peace, both with the trauma that had been blocking her and with her connection to nature and her own inner world. By the time we were through, her whole foundation seemed to have been completely reset; she had not only released the preoccupations of the day from her mind, but she walked with a noticeable new confidence and ease.

Taking time to turn inside out in this way can clear out and reopen our connection to our inner world. It's a valuable process, not just because it brings peace to a troubled part of our soul but because it also opens the way for our Heart Wisdom to flow freely. By establishing this connection, we can bring our life back into balance and realign our priorities. The results you will experience from this will be evident in your outer world. For example, your business might suddenly begin to grow, your profits might magically increase.

Or, as happened recently with Steve, one of my own clients, a business partner, who might have annoyed you no end, suddenly does a complete turnaround and starts being really friendly and cooperative for no discernible reason.

I had been working with Steve for a couple of months about something else entirely when he suddenly showed up one day looking exceptionally miserable. His energy seemed to be very low, and I could tell that something much more profound was going on with him than was usually the case.

When I asked Steve what was going on, he started telling me about a situation that he was experiencing with his business partner, Sean. Apparently, Steve and Sean's relationship had been deteriorating for some months, and for some reason, neither of them had felt able to confront the other about what was going on, and how they might be able to resolve things. Clearly, this was beginning to weigh very heavily on Steve. As I gently prompted him to tell me more, Steve explained that he and Sean hadn't really had any meaningful conversations in the last three months.

"So how do you do business?" I asked.

"Well, we both know pretty much what to do in our roles, and we just exchange e-mails every so often; but truly, it's not good. I don't know what to do or how things can change. We just don't communicate well. So I just leave it alone."

I then asked Steve if he wanted to explore this deeper and see if we could effect some change. Because, clearly, something did need to change!

As we moved through the process, Steve began to realize that he was afraid to be open and discuss his concerns with Sean for fear that Sean would quit the business, leaving Steve to run it on his own. As we went deeper into the source of this belief, it transpired that Steve's behavior had its roots in *his* own fear and beliefs around confrontation. He felt that if he ever raised any dissatisfaction or disagreed with Sean in any way, then his partner would leave, which would then screw up the business.

Upon tracking this belief farther inward, Steve came to realize that this was formed from his relationship with father. Steve's father had hated confrontation. Consequently, whenever Steve had brought something up as a child, his father would retreat from the conversation by either leaving the room, or leaving the house altogether.

When I questioned Steve as to what this behavior "meant" for him, he admitted that it had felt like betrayal on his father's part. Over the years, Steve's unconscious fear of "losing his father's love" had translated itself into an 'If-I-never-raise-anything-that-sounds-confrontational-I'll-never-give-people-reason-to-leave-me" belief system, which was now being played out in Steve's relationship with his business partner.

Once we identified the fear and unraveled the belief system, Steve was able to find peace within himself and relax both his mind and his body. However, the most amazing part was still to come. The next day Steve called me and told me that, "Out of the blue, without my even saying anything to Sean about the business, or what I had discovered doing your Heart Wisdom process, Sean had said that he'd had some great ideas for improving the business that he'd like to discuss!"

Our inner world is the place where magic and miracles happen. As we turn our attention inward and uncover the roots of our belief systems and behaviors, and learn to unravel them, we make space for something new to happen. As Steve discovered, transforming your life is not about having to learn a whole new way of being. It's simply about freeing yourselves from erroneous belief systems and the constraints that arise from them.

By navigating his inner world, Steve was able to connect with his Heart Wisdom. He was able to recognize the truth about and, thus, release an old belief system that had been constraining him. In the process, Steve had created space in his inner world for something else to happen, which then showed up in his outer world as a change in his relationship with Sean.

If you accept the premise that we are all one, then it's not such a far stretch to believe that in changing ourselves, we change the world around us. This has been brought home to me time and time again in my work with my clients. As we nurture our soul, all of our relationships, including our business relationships, benefit, because we are coming from a different place. We're coming from our heart and, therefore, from our authentic self.

Sadly it's more typical for people to approach their inner world in the same way that Susie had learned to approach nature when she was growing up. Like nature, the inner world feels like foreign territory full of potential hazards. The outer world seems safer because there are strict rules that govern what goes on and how we must behave in it, so we know where we stand—or at least we think we do. For example, societal conditioning has taught us to believe that if our bank account is empty, we should feel like a "failure." If our car is expensive, new and shiny, we can feel that we are a "success."

But "failure" and "success" are constructs of the mind, projected as judgments on our whole being, and out into the material world. Because of this, the outer world can be a useful guide to the state of our inner world; but to use it as a measure for our worth or whole being is a recipe for disaster. However, when we can remember what is truly fulfilling and connect to our core through Heart Wisdom, via our inner world, we realize that material things and people come and go, but "we"—the real, authentic us, with all the masks and status markers stripped away—remains.

The Truth isn't "out there"

The answers aren't "out there" for us to find and master. They are right here inside us, simply "waiting" for us to tap into them. The moment we truly recognize this is the moment that we finally come home to ourselves. The seeking is over.

Turning the World Inside-Right

There is so much magic and so many Divine gifts available to us in every moment, seeking us out if you will. Here is an example from my own personal experience of what can happen when you listen to your Heart Wisdom. About twelve years ago, I was living in Florida. Life was good. My business was good, I was in a passionate relationship. I was playing lots of great music. I had a great circle of friends! I was open. My life was flowing. My then girlfriend mentioned about going on this retreat into nature. From deep within me I felt this YES! It was an irresistible impulse that called me to more deeply explore my inner world.

I was on a mission to deepen my own relationship with nature and explore my inner world, so I signed up for a seven-day solo retreat called *Sacred Passage and the Way of Nature* in the Sangre de Cristo Mountains of southern Colorado. The intention behind this program was for each participant to experience the harmonization of their inner nature with external nature—to realize and recognize the value of their interconnectedness. In order for this to happen I had to retreat into solitude: for seven full days, I didn't see or speak to anyone. There was no cell phone. No e-mail. No books or sketch pad.

As you can imagine, the first few days were tough—decompression in its purest form. But as the days passed, I became more and more comfortable with the strange sounds and unfamiliarity of nature and those of my inner voice.

Each morning I would wake up in my tent, which was pitched right in the middle of the wilderness. There was nowhere to go. So I began a daily routine of relaxation and awareness exercises that included yoga, meditation and Qi Gong (a traditional Chinese medicine practice that coordinates different breathing patterns with a set of postures and movements). Next, I would eat a little and then walk around the area until I was ready to sit quietly outside my tent. Later in the day I would take a little nap, wake up and go through the same routine again. I repeated this same routine for three full cycles for each of the seven days. No distractions, just me, myself and "I."

Every evening I would meditate and watch the sun set behind the mountains. It was a beautiful way to end the day, and it certainly helped open me to nature, and my inner wonder at the magical order of the Universe. What fascinated me was how the sunset was so different each night because my senses became increasingly heightened as the days progressed.

On the fourth day as I looked out over the treetops to the emerging pink-and-orange glow, I felt as though I could see the tiniest detail of every leaf. Noises that I had barely noticed when I had first arrived were becoming clearer and more audible as the days passed—it was as though I could hear the ants crawling on the ground. I became aware of a faint sensation, a slight vibration in the air. As I stood perfectly still, all my senses extended, I became aware that what I was hearing and feeling was the vibration of life, the Universe, the interchange of information that passes in and between all living things.

HEART FACT

Human and animal heart cells, when placed together in a Petri dish, will beat in unison. But if you put different people's brain cells in a Petri dish together they are unable to communicate and they die.

During the last evening of my retreat, as I watched the sunset, I became aware that the vibrating sound, which was still present, appeared to be getting progressively closer, louder and more palpable—so close, it could have been a fly buzzing at the very edge of my ear. Then, all of a sudden, the sound went right into my head, and my whole world warped.

What was outside became inside, and what was inside seemed to be on the outside. The vibration was now emanating directly from the center of my head, dramatically shifting my entire energetic and sensory experience. Inner and outer nature had become one. Outer world had merged with inner world. This vibration, as I understood it, was the sound of the earth's electromagnetic field. I had literally harmonized with the earth!

Throughout that night and all through the next day this profound connection to nature expanded, gently wrapping around my heart, massaging it open. My attention settled into my heart as if finally arriving home after a long journey.

As the final morning dawned, I did one final practice, then packed up and began my journey back to base camp. As I began to walk, I noticed something astonishing: With each step, with each breath, I literally could feel the earth rise up in my body. My body was breathing and moving as part of the earth! I was moving and breathing from a deeper place, a connected place that seemed to be flowing from a deep openness within my body and within the earth itself! I felt suddenly energized by this dynamic current that seemed to be a direct line from my heart to the heart of the Universe. I could feel it filling me up and overflowing into every cell of my body.

In that instant I also felt an intensely clear and profound sense of belonging, both to the earth and to myself, the like of which I had never before experienced. Until that day I had always had a peculiar sense that I didn't truly belong. Yet, in that exquisite moment of harmonization with and between nature and me, it became apparent that the only reason I had lacked a sense of belonging was because I had been living out of harmony with my own inner nature, and, consequently, was cut off from my heart and the wisdom that flowed through it.

The effect of that experience on my life was wild! It was as though I had gone from black and white to full spectrum Technicolor—from screeching, ear-splitting static to the serenity of a perfectly tuned-in radio playing the sublime sounds of some heavenly choir. I'd been hearing that static all my life, and had never given it a second thought, assuming that it must be normal. Then I heard and experienced something else and realized how out of tune I was. Thanks to that harmonizing experience, what had seemed to be my true self turned inside out and simply swallowed up everything that I had mistakenly believed and tried to project onto the world. It made space for the real "me" to come through. Thank God!

From that time on there could be no going back. Since that experience, I have discovered that the more I truly allow myself to be myself and to bring whatever that is to the world's table, the more fulfillment and peace I can achieve, and therefore, the more fulfillment and peace I can create in the world around me. We all came here to contribute our gifts and to help evolve the world into a better place. However, we can't do that until we learn to access our inner world and tap into the wisdom of the heart to unleash those gifts so that they can finally flow freely through us. For our authentic self is that which we truly are. And who we truly are is the greatest gift we have to give to the world.

In order to give our gift, we must first turn ourselves inside out. By doing so, we begin the process of turning the whole world *inside right*.

Each day of that seven-day retreat took me farther and farther along on my healing journey. In my solitude, I took a quantum leap into my own inner world. From there, I could see how fragmented my daily life had been. Before that experience, I had pursued countless processes and experiences that had helped me journey deep into my heart and my inner world, but there was little or no integration. The moment the process or experience was over, I had always felt the magnetic pull, snapping me back into my head and the outer world to live the same old life again. This time it was different. This experience changed everything.

You'll be relieved to hear that retreating into nature for seven days isn't the only way to access your inner world and your Heart Wisdom! There are many alternative and simpler ways to reach this divine connection. But I do recommend regular visits to parks, beaches, mountain ranges and lakes, whichever is within reach of your home. And rather than spending this time in nature with a group of people gossiping about friends, family or the state of the world, do commit to spending some time in nature alone. Do this occasionally, but even better is to do it at least once a week, if not everyday! You will notice the difference in your energy, vibrancy and state of mind instantly, even if it doesn't give you the profound inner-outer, world-warping experience that I had!

The Breath as a Pathway
to Your Inner World

If you can't access nature on a regular basis, one of the easiest and most powerful ways to connect with your inner world is to do conscious breathing exercises—easy to do at home, in the office, the car or even on the subway. An amazing thing about breathing is that it seems so simple, yet the majority of people I have worked with have breathing patterns that are impaired in some way.

The most common problem is a reverse breathing pattern, meaning that when you inhale your abdomen goes in, rather than out, and when you exhale your abdomen goes out, rather than in. The correct pattern is just the opposite. When you inhale the abdomen should inflate and go out, and when you exhale it should deflate and go in. Take a look at your lower belly right now and see what is going on with your own breath. You assume your body is taking care of this for you, but if you're stressed, suffering a physical illness or caught up in your head, the chances are that your breathing will be back to front.

To correct this, place one or both hands on your abdomen. Take a nice deep breath right into the bottom of your lungs. What do you notice? When you inhale does your abdomen inflate or deflate or is it somewhere in the middle? Is it a strain to breathe deeply? What is the quality of the breath? How deeply does it go into your body? Can you even feel the bottom of your lungs? If your breathing pattern is not reversed, then your belly will become full as you inhale, and deflate as you exhale.

If this is the case, see how deeply you can bring the breath into your body. Can you breathe deeply into the lungs, bringing the air down through the heart, stomach and into your pelvis? With a very full breath, you'll feel the expansion, possibly accompanied by tingles, all the way down to your toes and up to your head as the oxygen freely circulates around the body. It feels expansive because the breath is not limited by the physiological and physical structures in your body.

If your breathing pattern is reversed, then your belly is deflating as you inhale, and inflating as you exhale. This isn't a sign of inferiority, I promise. But it is something that limits the amount of air you are taking in with each breath, and thus is constricting your ability to reach your inner world and your Heart Wisdom. It will also cause you a greater degree of stress and can have negative effects on the physical body. By following your breath into your body and finding these contractions you can do a "non-process release," meaning you can clear out some of your inner world clutter, just by releasing these contractions in your body.

This can be emotional. It may bring up very strong emotions, but it is really just a release. You are simply supporting your body's ability to unravel and unwind. To adjust your breathing, place your hands on the lower part of your abdomen, exhale completely and draw your abdomen muscles inward, or, in other words, draw your belly button back toward the spine. Now with laserlike focus, slowly inhale a deep long breath down through the top of your lungs, into the lower lungs, the stomach, the abdomen and then finally, into the bottom of your pelvis. Paying particular attention the breath as it passes through the abdomen allowing it to push the muscles outwards as the lungs fill fully with fresh air.

Take your time and really allow the breath to go as deeply into the pelvis as possible. Repeat this for at least three minutes. Notice how you feel when you are done. Are you in your head still? Do you feel calm or stressed? Notice if your heart feels more open or closed? The benefits of this breathing exercise are many. In addition to oxygenating the body and opening you to your inner world, this also helps open your physical inner space, clearing out toxins, blocked energy and emotions, opening the valves and cells as well as the heart.

We will return to the breath over and over again in this book. It is part of every exercise and integral to the practice section in the final part of the book. If you do all the exercises on these pages, by the end, you will be well on your way to making conscious breathing an integrated practice in your life. Your breathing is a profoundly important pathway into your inner world and a direct route to your Heart Wisdom, so developing this practice is like constructing your own superhighway that will lead you to your authentic self.

HEART WISDOM KEY NUMBER THREE

Using the Breath to Turn Your Attention Inward.

One of the easiest and most powerful ways to learn to focus inward is through conscious breathing exercises. This is a golden pathway into your inner world so developing this practice is like building your own superhighway to your true self.

By now you have already discovered your own breathing patterns. Now it is time to learn how to use the correct breathing technique to help you achieve and maintain that inward focus. If you would like me to guide you through this process you can go to the Heart Wisdom Web site (*www.heartwisdom.com*) and download the free MP3 recording I have made to guide you step by step through this exercise:

With your hands on the lower part of your abdomen, exhale completely and draw your abdomen muscles inward, or, in other words, draw your belly button back toward the spine.

Now with laser-like focus, inhale into the bottom of your pelvis and inflate your abdomen slowly, paying particular attention to allowing the breath to push the abdomen muscles out. Take your time and really allow the breath to go as deeply into the pelvis as possible. Allow it to inflate from the bottom of the pelvis up through the heart and into the throat.

Continue this consciously for three minutes. Not only are you shifting your breathing pattern to more deeply oxygenate the body but you are also retraining the muscles so that it becomes natural. By doing this exercise every day, for just three minutes at a time, you will begin to breath correctly, naturally and easily. You will also discover that you are much more attuned to your body's energy and your inner self.

CHAPTER FOUR

From Contraction to Expansion

There are only two ways to live your life.
One is as though nothing is a miracle.
The other is as though everything is a miracle.
— *ALBERT EINSTEIN*

What happens if you put a kink in a garden hose? The kink stops the flow of water through the hose and creates a buildup of pressure. Similarly, in the body, when you are open and hooked up to your Heart Wisdom you are part of the unfettered flow of the Universe. However, if you have any kinks, or "contractions" as I call them, that restrict or block the flow of energy, they will cause a buildup of tension. This, in turn, will impede or cut off your ability to receive the inherent wisdom of your heart. Just like the garden hose, once the kink is released, the path is clear for the energy to flow freely.

In our head-centered culture there are countless events, crises, traumas and obstacles that challenge our ability to stay open. These can create contractions of energy in the body, which we feel as tension. We're all contracted on some level, and we need to accept that fact. But when you start living from your heart, you will approach these challenges differently—creating less contraction—and have the tools to release the contractions in an instant.

Stress

Stress has been cited as the Number One contributory factor to premature aging and ill health. Unsurprisingly, it's also the Number One cause of contraction. We all know that certain types of stress can be bad for

HEART FACT
"The vascular system that supports your heart is over 60,000 miles long and could wrap around the earth twice."

us, but few of us appreciate fully the damaging effects that chronic stress has on our body, mind and spirit. For one thing, few of us are adept at recognizing many of the subtler symptoms of stress. These can be so vague—anxiety, mood swings, sleep disruption, headaches, gastric problems, loss of appetite, lowered sex drive, tiredness and lethargy—that it simply would not occur to us to relate them back to their true cause. For another, most of us have become so inured to juggling the many different aspects of our typical high-pressured modern-day lifestyles that we're not only unaware how deeply stressed we really are but we also have no idea that it's contracting our energy and cutting off our access to the very thing we need to make our life flow with grace and ease: our Heart Wisdom.

The horrifying truth is that most people are stressed beyond measure and are unaware of the debilitating effects it has on every area of their life; from physical health to relationships, from their ability to think clearly and be creative, or to simply enjoy life. Unfortunately, most people wait until they are in enough physical pain before they make a change, and some even don't do it then.

I am not suggesting that all stress is bad. There is good stress as well—the kind of stress that is motivating and supportive, that drives us to take positive action on some project or unresolved issue in our life, or gives us the impetus to get things done. But that is not what I am talking about here. What concerns me the most about stress, because I see it so often in my clients, are the subtler, more insidious effects of chronic stress and how it congests the way we think, feel, communicate and interact with others, and how it blocks our ability to create, manifest and attract great things into our lives.

When we are stressed, a common default pattern is for us to go straight into our head to find refuge and escape from feeling the discomfort. Indeed, on the surface, this would seem like a good approach, but in actuality, it is a horrible strategy. Systematically avoiding stress creates a resistance to our own natural self-corrective mechanism. When we don't manage our stress it accumulates and takes root in the body. When we avoid it, it just grows wild and, consequently, becomes more difficult to remove. Just imagine the difference between removing a newly planted seedling from the ground versus the root system of a 100-year-old tree. Obviously, it would be easier to remove the seedling. So clearing stress needs to happen regularly in order to decongest our inner world. It is a good idea to start with the more recently planted seedlings, then move on to deep excavation. (But we'll get to that part later.)

One of the most visible examples of unmanaged stress can be seen in those people who just can't seem to sit still. They're either constantly jiggling their foot, pacing around, or tapping their fingers on any surface they can find. And, by the way, if mention of this rubs an edge for you and you find yourself reacting to what I'm saying, please note that's a good thing! I'm not saying this to upset you or to be antagonistic; I'm saying it because anything that causes a strong reaction in us is worthy of further investigation. Instant recoil is a protective mechanism. It's the mind's way of saying, "don't go there, don't look at that, you're not going to like what you find if you do."

But that's the very time when we do need to stay present, to go within and find what it is about that person, thing or behavior that bugs us so much, and to do something about it. Invariably, we'll find that it is not the thing, person or behavior we don't like; it's the *meaning* we have attached to it.

Remember, awareness (becoming aware) is the first step in the process of transformation. The more self-aware we become, the more opportunities we create to *choose* our responses. We can choose to move through life on automatic pilot, with no control over our reactions, and no understanding of what or even whose tapes or programs are "pulling our strings." Or we can choose to free ourselves to move into a more conscious, centered, heart-connected place. From that place, it becomes easy and natural to initiate the positive changes we want and need to make in order to live authentically and joyfully.

This reminds me of another of my Florida experience. This time I was attending my first "rebirthing" session with my then girlfriend. Rebirthing uses a specific method of breathing to liberate suppressed energy, stress and patterning within the body. The idea is to release the old patterning and literally give birth to your liberated self. Chris Retzler, a renowned rebirther from England, explains it beautifully: "Rebirthing is a healing process that engages with the mind, the body and the spirit to cleanse away toxic patterns of being and facilitate new, healthy and fulfilling goals and choices. The core practice of Rebirthing is a breathing technique; the core metaphor is the rebirth of the personality through the integration of suppressed experience."

When the process started, I remember thinking, "I wonder if this is going to work for me. I don't see how this is going to happen." Then I started focusing on my breath, which took me out of my head. Within a few minutes, I was astonished to find that my hands were clenched, my body was contracting in pain and tears were pouring down my face. A few moments later, I was curled up in the fetal position, crying like a baby. All this just from just breathing! Wow! What I discovered was that the pain was coming from repressed and suppressed emotions, and energy. It was deep core tension that had gotten trapped in my body and built up, layer upon layer, over the years.

The most significant part of this catharsis was that I became aware that love was the only thing that mattered. Nothing else seemed to make sense—nothing anyone said or did, nothing I thought about or tried to think about. The only thing that brought any ease to my painful body, my world, my being, was love —the love and care that came from the support team and my girlfriend. It was the pure presence of love and genuine caring. I experienced the bare bones truth of it all: when all is said and done, nothing matters but love, the love that can be accessed through the wisdom of the heart. Yes, other things play a part in our fulfillment, but as expressed in the immortal lyrics of Robert Hunter, "Without love in the dream it will never come true." This was another experience that changed my life forever.

Understand that when you experience stress, you are actually, on some level, holding on to it. It's similar to holding a pen in your hand. It takes energy and effort to hold the pen. After a while if you keep holding it, you will tend not to notice as much, and maybe even forget about it, at least for a while. It's the same with stress or tension. Some event happens in your life, your body contracts as a defense mechanism to protect itself, and on some level the body is still holding on to that "shock." For as long as the shock is there, the body is not open, your energy is constricted and your heart cannot access its inherent wisdom. What is interesting to note is that animals instinctually will retreat into solitude after a traumatic experience and tremble and shake in order to release the shock. It seems we have a lot to learn from our animal friends.

Energetic Integrity

As you begin to explore the issues that might be causing you stress, it is essential to be listening for where the "in" is. The "in" is the place where you can literally feel the weakening of the energy field (your own or another person's). This is what I call Energetic Integrity (EI): the quality of the field of energy that emanates from and surrounds the physical body. When stress or a constriction is present, the EI is often weakened; the vibrancy is low and its reach is limited. In contrast, when someone is either managing their stress in a healthy manner, or completely stress-free and are connected to their Heart Wisdom, their EI is strong and radiant, and emanates fully around them.

We've all seen individuals who seem to have such an amazing presence that people's eyes seem riveted to them. These are the people that often seem to exude some kind of special energy or aura. We may not necessarily see it or feel it, but we definitely notice it, and that leaves us wondering, "Who is that person, and what special quality do they have that draws everyone's attention?"

When the body is holding on to something unresolved, it will automatically readjust itself to accommodate this. The simplified version is that in the same way that a river will take the path of least resistance by flowing around a rock that is in the middle of it, so too will the body compensate by finding a way to accommodate itself to the tension, or disruption in its field, caused by stress of an unresolved issue. However, it takes a lot of energy for the body to compensate in this way. As a result, the flow of energy through the body will be restricted, which in turn comprises its integrity. The greater the contraction in the body, the more energy is required to compensate.

As time passes, and this holding pattern becomes more deeply entrenched, the body will begin to organize itself differently. There is a domino effect as one piece (or system) is affected and it begins to impact all the others. Eventually, this process will begin to double back on itself, and overlay pattern upon pattern upon itself. So when you bury an issue (consciously or unconsciously), or let the contractions build up by trying to "stuff them under the rug," you really are doing just that. It is very important to realize that the more you bury, the more you reinforce and strengthen your contractions, and the heavier your emotional baggage becomes.

Consequently, your EI weakens, which in turn increases your susceptibility to stress and disease. As your vibrancy diminishes, your energy field shrinks and your spirit starts to feel as if it's fading or thinning. You may recall hearing yourself or someone else say, "I just don't feel like myself today" or "I just feel so disconnected." Your EI is like a thermometer. That's why some psychics, energy healers and intuitives like me are able to tap in to what is going on for people and recognize those who are in need of healing.

Stuffing down your pain might help you feel better for a while; however, your suffering will always resurface and come "knocking on your door" again until you get to the core of the issue. You must heed the call of your innate intelligence/wisdom. This festering "core issue" is the root of chronic conditions. If you never reach the root, the condition will persist and continue to manifest in one form or another. There is no greater reward than your wellbeing. Reaching the root of your core condition is the gateway to your liberation, as Rose, one of my clients discovered after coming to me with the complaint of feeling stressed, depressed and emotionally repressed.

As we began exploring her situation, Rose shared that she didn't know how to deal with her parents or what to say to them. They were very controlling and it was freaking her out. When we talked about how she thought her parents viewed her life, I intuitively sensed her EI weaken. That was the "in," and it was clear to me that she was still looking for approval from her parents. We then tracked the energy in her body. She began feeling twinges of pain in her heart and a deep sadness. Then she dropped a little deeper into a place of loneliness, profound loneliness. I supported her to stay open and just feel. The most important thing was to not to try to get through it, but to open deeper and to feel the physical sensations and the emotions attached to them completely. Remember, the body knows how to heal itself; our only job is to stay present with it and allow the healing to happen!

HEART FACT
"Your heart is a powerful organ. It can produce enough energy in one hour to lift a 2000 lb car three feet off the ground!"

As Rose turned her attention inward, I intuited that something had contracted within her around the age of three. While staying open, I then invited her to connect with herself as a three-year-old child. Rose's face seemed to crumple like a little child's. "I just feel so sad," she said.

"Do you think you could be okay with just being sad?" I gently asked her. When she didn't answer, I then said, "I want you to realize there is a part of you that is not allowing it to be okay for you to be sad. Where did you learn that? Being sad is a part of you, and every part of you needs to be loved and cherished. Would you be willing to just be with the sadness for a little while?"

As I watched Rose struggle with the memory of her three-year-old self's pain, it became clear that she was trying to fix the sadness. This is not an uncommon response. It stems from the belief that there is something wrong with our feelings, which can then get interpreted as "there is something wrong with me."

Trying to fix her pain was another core pattern that emerged for Rose as a contraction. This is deeply rooted in the old masculine paradigm, and comes from her role as a woman surviving in a male-dominated world. Men traditionally like to fix things. They are doers. This is not good or bad, it just is. Somewhere along the way, Rose had acquired the belief that there was something wrong that needed to be fixed—namely her! She then went on to live from this place, trying to fix herself (and others), always feeling that "something is wrong or missing, therefore I must be broken."

Throughout our session, Rose kept expressing that she "just wanted to feel love." The very fact that she 'wanted to feel love' presupposed that "love was missing" from Rose's life. Her mind then interpreted this as "I am unlovable, I must be broken," which fed right back into the loop of Rose's core issue. No wonder her body was contracting, creating stress and pain! When we believe that something is true, we are unconsciously impelled to prove ourselves right. So long as Rose *believed* that she was broken and needed to be fixed, her unconscious need to be right would drive her to keep on creating situations in her life that needed fixing. Consequently her search for love continued, endlessly.

During the session with Rose she revealed that her biological father had left home when she was three years old, which had devastated her mother. From that point on, Rose's mother had begun to withhold her own love, and consequently Rose developed the belief that "there must be something wrong with her." There was no Daddy, no one to take care of things, to take care of *her* or "fix" things, as men do. When her Dad left, it registered that love had gone away, and she now had to find it. A parent's role is not to "fill" their child with love, but rather, to support their child to stay open to love. For love already exists! When Rose's father left and her mother abandoned her emotionally, there was no one left to help her remain open to love, to remind her that love was all around her and within her! Consequently, Rose had unconsciously closed her own heart.

The subconscious pattern Rose had been continually playing out in her life was that she was looking for the Daddy who had left her. Going deeper, we can also see that she was just desperately looking for something that would help her stay open to love, to reconnect with the source of love within her, her own heart and its wisdom, as opposed to constantly chasing love and trying to track it down in her outer world.

This was a deeply cathartic process for Rose. Once she began to understand what had been driving her behavior, waves of sadness, anger and loneliness rose within her. Encouraging her to stay present with the process and just bear witness to the emotions and feelings flooding through and out of her body, I was able to guide Rose farther into the presence of her true self. As she gradually moved deeper, and allowed herself to open up more, she was able to release all the pent-up stress and tension that had been blocking her recognition of her true essence and her connection to her Heart Wisdom. After many minutes of allowing the unwinding process to occur, Rose was finally able to let go of her suffering and "restore" the inherent love that she had always had difficulty "finding" outside herself, and reconnect to the truth that resided within her Heart's Wisdom.

Once you have tasted "The Great Love" that resides in your heart center, you realize that the love we all spend so much time and energy seeking is right here inside us all the time. I remember once hearing that "Everything is love. And everything that is not love is just love in a confused state." Love is. Love is all there is. And the heart is the crown jewel of your life! In terms of transformation, the heart is the alpha and the omega—the beginning with no end.

Releasing and Restoring

Rose had spent her entire life seeking, all the while believing that even if she found it, she couldn't keep it, because she wasn't worthy, she felt broken. Nonetheless, love was there all the time. All Rose had to do was to open herself up to releasing the contractions stored within her physical, mental and emotional bodies, and restore her connection to her Heart Wisdom.

You can do it, too. Start by noticing when something is bothering you. Become aware of your Energetic Integrity, feel for the contractions in the body and allow your body to unwind. You must allow yourself to feel whatever you are feeling. As you let go and allow yourself to feel deeper into yourself, you will open to a force of intelligence, that will allow your spirit, your innate wisdom to be revealed. And in that embrace you allow it to "take care of you," to heal and balance you.

I am repeating the word "allow" intentionally here. *Allow* this process. This is the heart of trust —trusting that the Divine is guiding you in a beneficial direction. It helps to practice it often, as this will support and sustain your ability to stay open. The great fear so many people feel deep down inside comes from feeling disconnected from the source that lives and breathes within us. We have forgotten the primary force that nourishes, truly nourishes our existence. We have literally lost the feeling of being "taken care of," and our souls are desperately seeking this nourishment.

I teach a very simple practice to all of my clients when they first come to me that helps them identify their contractions. Over and over again it has proved invaluable in helping them to cultivating awareness, opening their body, and freeing it from all tensions and modes of contraction. Before you can tap in to the subtler energies within, you must first learn to assist your body in realizing that you have a choice in your ability to manage physical tension, emotional pain and stress, and in letting it go.

Before we move on to learning how to identify contraction, I'd just like to share one more story about one of my clients and her experience of this practice. It was a beautiful California day, so Sharon and I decided we would walk on the beach together. As we were walking, I couldn't help noticing how out of balance Sharon was. Literally, her left shoulder was about three inches closer to her left ear than her right shoulder was to her right ear. When I mentioned it to her, she said her shoulder had been like that for about six months, and it bothered her because it looked strange. It also ached constantly, and she felt drained of energy. This was affecting Sharon's career because she was a model. The way her body looked and how she felt about it had a direct impact on whether or not she worked.

She asked me if I knew of any massage techniques that would help her shoulder. She then began to tell me about all of the different theories she had for why it was like that. These ranged from an old snowboarding injury resurfacing, to carpal tunnel, to a "hunch" about something!" All of her theories made sense to her, but none of them helped solve the problem with her shoulder.

I thanked her for her stories and let her know that I didn't need to know any more about why she thought her shoulder was locked up. As she spoke I read her field and got a sense of her EI. It was then that I suggested to her that there might be another way that I could help her, if she was open to it.

I explained that actually, she didn't need to know *why* it was locked up. I had an "intuitive hunch" that the only question she needed to focus on was this: "Is there any reason why you can't just drop your shoulder?" She could move her head, her legs, her arms; she could jump up and down, raise her hand and kick up her heels. Why couldn't she just choose to drop her shoulder?

Of course, she couldn't think of any reason that didn't involve an irrelevant story. As I continued to read her field, I could see that the contraction was rooted in her mind. Somewhere within her psyche, Sharon was holding a limiting belief, and it was manifesting as a physiological symptom.

As we continued walking, I told Sharon to bring her attention to her shoulder, to focus and breathe and let go while asking herself that question, "Is there any reason why I just can't drop my shoulder?" She was skeptical, so I suggested she try it on her own, at her own pace in the privacy of her own home.

After a month of doing the exercises I had recommended, Sharon's shoulder dropped to its proper position became level with her other shoulder and the pain subsided. She was thrilled. By resting her attention on this shoulder and breathing into it as a daily practice, she allowed her body's healing power to take care of the problem. Her shoulder had dropped, without having to resort to pills, shots or massage.

Sharon had not had to rely on anything external, other than a little advice and encouragement. Now, two years later, her shoulders are level most of the time. But when her life falls out of balance and stress pushes her into a mode of contraction, her shoulder creeps right back up to her ear, just like an alarm sounding to remind her about breathing and "taking care of" her soul, her body and her connection to her heart wisdom.

HEART WISDOM KEY NUMBER FOUR

Finding Your Contraction

I suggest you read through this exercise several times to familiarize your-self with it before getting started. Alternatively, you can go to the Heart Wisdom Web site (*www.heartwisdom.com*) and download the free MP3 recording I have made to guide you step by step through this exercise.

• Begin by bringing your attention to the top of your head and, like an X-ray machine, start scanning slowly down through your body, paying particular attention to any places where you feel aware that you might be holding some tension, or as if something is "stuck" there. Allow your senses to be your guide. As soon as you sense you are feeling something, just hold your awareness there for several moments. You will notice that just by bringing your attention and awareness there, the tension will start to release itself naturally. It is like bringing a candle into a dark room. The light (of awareness) "disperses" any darkness or density.

• Next, start doing the breathing exercise that I outlined at the beginning of this chapter.

• Scan your muscles and breathe – identify your contractions

• Scan your bones and breathe – identify your contractions, release and restore.

• Scan your eyes, your neck, your jaw, and your torso, all the while remembering to keep breathing and identifying your contractions. Then release and restore.

- As you perform these simple techniques over and over, you will notice a relaxing, a recovering and a release taking place. This practice will help restore your body to a healthy state and restore your soul to its rightful place—connected to your heart rather than your head. It will also replace stress with love, unrest with peace, confusion with clarity and exhaustion with an infusion of energy.

CHAPTER FIVE

Releasing Negative Beliefs and Emotions

*The moment you have in your heart
this extraordinary thing called love and feel the depth,
the delight, the ecstasy of it, you will discover
that for you the world is transformed.*

—*KRISHNAMURTI*

Feeling your emotions fully is the gateway to freedom, but suppressing your emotions is a mode of contraction that will obviously affect your heart and your ability to tap into your Heart Wisdom. Most people were never taught about emotional health; yet, it plays an essential role in experiencing optimal health. As a result, we are overrun with debilitating blockages that inhibit our expression of emotions and directly affect our levels of fulfillment, joy and creativity.

The Role of Emotions

Have you ever noticed how a child seems to have boundless energy? You may have heard someone or yourself say, "Boy, that child wears me out." Why does a child have so much energy? For the most part, children express their emotions the minute they feel them. If it hurts, they cry or yell. If they are upset, they let you know. When they are happy, they

HEART FACT

Your aorta is the largest artery in your body and is about the size of a garden hose. Your capillaries are so tiny that it would take ten of them to equal the size of a human hair. Yet, both work together to see to it that every cell of your body receives oxygen and nourishment.

laugh. When they get scared, they scream, yell, cry or even laugh. A child who is not subject to restrictive conditioning and who has been supported to express themselves will fully develop "emotional vitality."

Emotional vitality is the healthy development of what's known as the emotional body or emotional system. Emotional vitality shows up in the EI of your energetic field. When you are emotionally open you are like an unkinked garden hose. The energy of life can flow fully and freely through the body, continuously nourishing and fueling it.

This emotional vitality can be developed and restored in the body, no matter what your age or prior experiences. Emotional vitality is directly linked to anti-aging as well as stress and pain management. Emotions play an important role in keeping us healthy, too. When you hold them in, stuff them down, refuse to get angry, sorrowful, upset or even joyful, then you are severely compromising the health and functioning of your body. Emotions, being energy, need to move, they need to go somewhere.

If you direct your emotions inward, rather than outward, then eventually something will combust. Suppressed emotions build up as "negative" energy in the body, stagnant, rotting feelings that were never set free. You can only imagine the effect this has on your physical health and wellbeing. When you get this kind of emotional buildup, it's like rush hour on the freeway. Accessing your Heart Wisdom with all of this "stuff" blocking the way is inevitably challenging, if not virtually impossible. So, in order to get through to the wisdom of the heart, you must first understand how harmful holding back really is, and discover how to release any emotions that are trapped from your past.

But, first let's go a little deeper into the nature of emotions. Emotions = energy in motion. Emotions are not good or bad. They are just energy, and they are part of a self-regulating system in the body. Within this system each emotion serves a vital function to maintain optimal health. For example, anger, which is one of the most powerful and intense emotions, serves to ground the energy in the body and support your sense of safety and stability. Grounding is essential, and understanding how to stay grounded is powerful. This is how financial awakening coach Paul Lemon explains it:

Consider a two-wire electrical system. One of the wires is hot and the other grounds the system. When you flip the switch, the grounding wire communicates back to the source what is really happening in the system—for example, the switch has been flipped and energy needs to flow. When the energy is circulating in an open healthy system, the switch is flipped and the "circuitry" is connected and grounded. There is juice to fuel and inspire our lives. When the system becomes short circuited or ungrounded, the flow of the energy is obstructed and we don't get the juice we need where we need it.

In the case of anger, when the energy of anger gets backed up, we tend to get a little crazy, which is an excess, or backup, of energy in the head. And if it is short-circuiting out (leaking) through the head, then we can feel spacey.

To keep the energy flowing without constriction, it is important to feel everything—to unblock the fullness of your energy! If you were not fully supported and encouraged to feel and express your feelings and energies as a child (or even as an adult), there is a contraction of energy, which can manifest as tension, negative emotions or shutting down in certain situations. When you are shut down and holding tension in your body you think differently. It is very difficult to be creative and loving when you are stressed out and tense.

So many of us carry our emotional baggage around like an eight-ton barge attached to our backs. We bring it everywhere we go. We've heaped so much on top that we don't even know what's there anymore. We just know that it's heavy and slows us down. What if we could just release it all and be forever free of it? Conventional psychotherapy asks us to climb on board the barge and pick up every individual piece of trauma, sadness, disappointment and betrayal and "talk" about it. To hold it up to the light, look at it from every angle and not put it down until we know what it is, why it hurt and what impact it's had on our lives. For some, that barge is so jam-packed full of junk, that "talking" our way through it wouldn't just take years, but lifetimes!

If you ask me, that's way too much work for way too little result! We don't want to be processing our entire life when the point of even being here is to enjoy every moment we can. Just like releasing tension in the body, releasing emotions can be a matter of focusing attention, choosing to let go and trust that your Heart Wisdom to show you the way. Emotions are there to give you guidance, to show you what "feels right" and what doesn't. When tapping into your emotions, in conjunction with your Heart Wisdom, you can become powerfully discerning about the situations, people, opportunities and risks that are presented to you in your life. If you ignore the emotions and ignore the cues, you ignore information that is trying to tell you something.

The Harm of Holding Back

Another problem is that most people hold back their emotions, which means they restrict the flow of energy through the body and inevitably the heart (the gateway to the soul and the source of love). Thus, in essence they are holding back love! Again, "everything is love, and everything that is not love is just love in a confused state." No matter what, it all comes down to love. As the great Louis Armstrong sang, "Friends shaking hands, saying how do you do, all they're really saying is I love you."

It is by feeling fully, experiencing all the emotions and not by holding back, that our lives, our path, our gifts can come into clear vision. The next problem is that we hold our emotions back because they are painful. Pain is not fun! Though pain is a part of life, holding onto pain, holding back how we feel, causes suffering and makes the heart contract. When the pain is not released, the heart remains guarded, contracted, un-open. What should be a flow of energy becomes stagnant. The contractions of past, unresolved experiences restrict the flow of love through your heart, through your body and into your life. These contractions come from circumstances, beliefs and experiences about love, relationships and yourself.

Many people also hold back because they think it is protecting them in some way from a perceived vulnerability. People rationalize that holding back how they feel is going to somehow pay off in dividends. It doesn't. This is a distortion. Holding back your emotions restricts your energy, and even worse, it creates a negative imprint in your energy field and in the relationship or experience where you have chosen to suppress yourself.

If you engage people in this way, don't think for a moment it will somehow get easier. This is especially true if you are beginning a new relationship, job or partnership. If we meet someone and open to their love, the heart might open for a while, but then the old pattern returns and we start holding back.

If we start worrying that our lover might withdraw their love or the situation might change, our attention and energy will immediately return to the feeling of hurt that we've retained, to the "yucky" stuff that prevents us from remaining open to the beauty of love, to the joy and fulfillment and happiness we desire. Now you have imprinted how you will deal with emotions that come up in the relationship, but it is unsustainable.

As intimacy develops, at some point, you will have to clear that imprint or the relationship will not survive. Explore how this feels for a moment. Is that how you ultimately want to be in relationship—stuck in some kind of emotional check? If not, then why start that way! You will only have to backtrack in some covert mission of damage control. But, what is important to remember is that the "yucky" stuff is still you on some level. It comes from your own choices, patterns, conditioning and karma. These are your patterns, your stuff. It's your responsibility or, better yet, your *opportunity* to liberate and open to your Heart Wisdom!

When it all comes down to it, what really holds people back from expressing their feelings and loving fully is a program of fear. It might be a fear of rejection, or that your feelings won't be reciprocated, or that you aren't good enough or that you don't have enough of something to keep the other person interested in you.

For example, if as a child you did something your parents didn't like (i.e., wrote on the walls, stole a candy bar, bashed your sibling over the head with a stick!) and they "withdrew" their love, you may well have developed a pattern that suggests that if you do something someone doesn't like, or approve of, then they may withdraw their love.

So what then happens is that you have this unconscious fear program running that people will withdraw their love if you do something they disapprove of, and then you start doing things to please others to get their love or approval. Past injuries like these cause the heart and emotions to shut down. Typically the following are what hold people back from being emotionally honest, also known as "emotional honesty":

- Worrying about how your "truth" will be received, or not received;
- Being concerned that it will create confrontation and conflict;
- Being scared that your requests will provoke anger in the other person;

- Thinking you will not be liked or loved;
- Feeling that you will look bad, or be perceived as bad;
- Not trusting that your feelings are valid.

It is important to understand that when you are holding back, you are rooted in a dynamic of "giving to get": that you should only give your love and emotional honesty when you are guaranteed to get the same in return. This is not Heart Wisdom. This is conditional love. This is a head game. Your head is playing fear games on you, allowing the fearful mind chatter to drown out the pleading desires of the heart for love, love and more love, free expression, emotion, elation, ecstasy and joy. When you live from the wisdom of your heart, you give love for no other reason than to share love, offering an unconditional gift, with no attachments. Or as I heard it put one time, "love doesn't love for a reason."

I once worked with a client called Catherine, who had become so used to holding back her emotions that it was beginning to influence every aspect of her life. Her posture was rigid, and there was a strain in her voice. She would talk quickly and immediately jump to intellectualizing. Intuitively, I could sense an energetic pattern of her redirecting her attention out of her heart and into her head. This was most noticeable when she spoke. Empathically, I could also feel the strain in her heart and an immense sadness that was welled up inside of her.

During our sessions, she would come to the edge of letting go, the edge of bravery and courage, and then she would stop cold in her tracks! She'd start talking and fidgeting in an attempt to avoid going over that edge. I say, "attempt," because that "doesn't flush" in the context of this work. So every time she tried to avoid the "truth"—her emotional truth—I would continue to bring her back to the moment, the moment of what was really happening with her emotions underneath.

And what was really happening was that her body wanted to release and let go of the deep emotional tension and suffering that had been building up within her, year after year. She would continue to avoid it because she thought it was just too painful to deal with it. The reality is that, in the end, not dealing with the pain is far more painful!

Eventually, with lots of support and encouragement, Catherine felt safe enough to stop holding back. When she finally let go, her entire body began to tremble as she released all those years of pent-up emotion. I kept supporting her to breathe and simply allow her body to release everything that it had been holding onto. Just as I said, "It's probably going to get a little more intense," she started to release the energy on all levels. She experienced full body tremors as the tears coursed uncontrollably down her cheeks. It took several long minutes to clear everything that had been locked up inside Catherine for so many years. But once she had released it all, the difference in her was palpable. You could literally see in her face that years of stress and aging had suddenly fallen away from her.

Although this kind of release can be intense (remember there is another way—releasing your emotions every day in every way!) the results are incredibly beneficial. Within weeks of our letting-go session, Catherine reported experiencing a profound sense of peace and freedom within her body that she hadn't experienced in years. Catherine's experience clearly reveals that holding back really isn't fun. And it truly serves no one. Letting rip with one's emotions might feel a little scary at first, but if you can just stay with it, you will soon experience a lightness of being and a joy that will leave you wanting more. Expressing your emotions can become "addictive," though! Some of the incredible rewards that my clients have experienced when expressing their truth include:

- A feeling of being relaxed, open and free—available for whatever presents itself to them in the moment, rather than being concerned with matters passed.
- A sense of being temporarily exhausted. This comes from the release of "cellular fatigue" because the person opened up and connected with areas they had been unconsciously holding for a long time. The exhaustion soon left and was replaced by vibrant energy.
- They encountered pain and tension that was hidden or suppressed in the body as a coping strategy, coupled with a lack of understanding of what was happening. After the "release" the pain dissipated and they were, often for the first time in years, able to experience the joy of an unencumbered body, without tension, pain or suffering.
- A rejuvenated libido, as well as a renewed sense of passion, sensitivity and bodily pleasure!
- They cultivated an intuitive and strong connection with their inner self.

- They were able to create the conditions and a clear path for easy connection to their Heart Wisdom and the Divine guidance therein.

Where we tend to get stuck with the pain and fear that surround our emotions is when we make them about another other person. We say, "Someone hurt me," or "they won't love me" when what's really happening is we feel hurt. And because we don't know how to deal with the hurt we make up a story about what we believe they will do, or won't do. By doing this, we skirt responsibility and miss a massive opportunity. We are colluding with an old paradigm of victimization," which causes us to stay stuck in the fear and pain. This can be healed naturally in time. But if we don't track the blocked hurt emotions and unwind, or release, them we haven't, and can't, and won't really heal anything deeply and completely.

HEART FACT

The muscles in your heart are so powerful that they can squirt blood up to 30 feet in a single beat.

Breaking Open

Heartbreak is really an opportunity to allow yourself to open to the source of your happiness and nourishment. The opportunity exists for your heart to "break open" to a greater love, to deeper feeling, to Heart Wisdom. I remember one client who was resistant to allowing the fullness of her emotions, to fully feeling the intensity of her experience. She was holding on and resisting falling apart. I told her it was okay to fall apart, that falling apart was good, and that this was a very good place to fall apart. We all need to fall apart from what we think is happening and who we think we are, for this is the only way to fall open to what is truly happening and who we truly are.

A key to working with this is to feel where you are shut down or are holding back emotions in your body—to feel where the energy is getting stuck and allow the body to unwind. But the master key is not to *try to get through it*, but to *go into it*—to penetrate the heart of the contraction, to unwind, to excavate and to release the core tension that is causing the symptoms you are experiencing. The unwinding will open the space for something new to happen. Remember, the body knows what to do and where it is going. There is an innate wisdom that always brings it back into balance, back into flow!

Breaking open is about releasing the emotions that are trapped. You are releasing tensions in your body by conscious choice. These may be tensions that you have been holding for years, but letting them go can be very simple: focusing your attention, breathing and letting go. It helps if someone else can hold the space of unconditional love for you so you can share the depth of your darkness, shame, guilt or pain.

If someone cannot hold that space, you or he/she may get triggered and take the emotional release personally, and/or react and get caught up in it. The space will then feel unsafe, and you will revert to holding back. You will likely pull back and shut down on some level because you don't feel safe or taken care of. Some crucial elements need to be established for you to explore the release of your emotions with another person. You must:

- Open to a place beyond conscious awareness. In this way, you can attain a greater understanding of who you are and truly expand your consciousness;
- Develop profound trust in the "greater" intelligence of life;
- Be willing to let go of who you think you are and be willing to open to and experience who you really are;
- Learn how to understand your conditioning and become conscious of your core story;
- Take full responsibility for your life and your contribution to any conflict or dysfunction going forward;
- Remember not to take yourself too seriously. Seriously enough to stay engaged in the process/in the game, but not too seriously that you constrict the flow of life and your joy;
- Cultivate profound self-acceptance and learn the art of self-love;
- Learn true forgiveness—not as an intellectual gesture but as a deep energetic and emotional opening, understanding and offering of love and a movement of Divine depth and penetration.

As you begin this process of release, it might feel a little scary. But remember, it is as simple as feel, focus, breathe and release (let go and allow). Also realize that the process itself is not scary; it is what you are holding onto as well as the unknown that lies just beyond the holding on that feels scary. The art of emotional release is to continuously track the energy through your body, on a multidimensional level, taking into account the tensions or "contractions" on an emotional, mental and physical level, so you can completely unwind the energy and fully open your body, from the inside out, to the wisdom of your heart.

Fearless Forgiveness

Forgiveness is the final stage in emotional liberation, and it is one of the most powerful vehicles to facilitate openness and emotional release. Forgiveness gives you the opportunity to let go of what is weighing you down, and it loosens up the energy between you and that to which you are attached. Not forgiving is a poison that pollutes your soul. In plain terms, an unwillingness to forgive actually hurts the person who is withholding forgiveness more than the person who is not being forgiven. When you are unwilling to forgive, three things occur:

1. You are holding yourself in an unfulfilling place.

2. You are enabling another to remain in an unfulfilling place.

3. In your refusal to forgive, you are holding emotional energy in your body that gets stored as tension. It lingers and festers and compounds, layer upon layer, over time.

Sometimes it is challenging to forgive someone who you feel has hurt or harmed you in some way. I remember hearing the renowned Rabbi Harold Kushner lament, [in this case] "think of forgiveness as being not willing to hold on to a specific person or situation any longer." For example, think of a situation you are currently involved in where there is something unresolved with another person. As you think about them, notice how you feel. Where are you feeling it in your body? Remember, if you are feeling it in your body, it is your stuff, your responsibility.

HEART WISDOM KEY NUMBER FIVE

Releasing Blocked Emotions

Releasing, unwinding and dissolving "negative" and blocked emotions are essential in the practice of Heart Wisdom. It is one of the keys that will unlock your unique light, your incredible gifts and the experience of living the life you both deserve and desire.

For this exercise you'll need a piece of paper or journal and pen. I'd like you to identify three emotional truths that you have avoided sharing, even though you really wanted to communicate them. Then write down the names of the three different people to whom you wished to communicate these emotional truths but didn't. Write down why you think you did not communicate your truth. What held you back? What fears got in the way? What "truth" do you need to communicate to them?

Now I want you to take each emotional truth, one by one, and examine why you think you did not communicate it by doing the following practice:

1. Start with a few minutes of conscious breathing.

2. Soften your attention into your heart.

3. Open your eyes softly, then read the first truth.

4. As you read it feel where you feel it in your body and notice what thoughts, emotions and sensations come up for you.

5. Allow yourself to feel the mind-body-spirit impact of the truth fully for a few minutes or until it feels complete for the moment.

6. Do the same with the other two.

7. When you are finished, write in your journal or on a piece of paper about your experience.

8. Bold and Bonus step: After you have done this release process, if you feel still unresolved with the person to whom you wanted to express this truth, call them and share how your felt about what happened. If possible, schedule a time to connect in person. Remember to just be yourself and share from the heart. Be gentle with yourself. It takes courage to speak your truth from the heart.

CHAPTER SIX

Engaging the Heart

Love is the only way to live that is not insane.
—*MYKANOS, FROM WILD NIGHTS BY DAVID DEIDA*

We all know people who seem really committed to quitting smoking, only to fall completely "off the wagon" the moment something stressful occurs in their life.

How does this happen?

It's easy to do because the "patterning" of that particular habit is so strong that it becomes deeply ingrained in the body and psyche. Something upsetting happens, cigarettes have always made you feel better, so in that moment you automatically reach for them again. Yes, nicotine is a known addictive substance, but it's actually often not the cigarette itself that provides the fix; it's the meaning your mind has ascribed to the behavioral ritual of smoking—or sex, or shopping, or whatever an individual's particular habit might be.

Smoking, sex and shopping are three of the most common examples of how deeply ingrained mental patterns control our behavior. Other conditions, which I call "veils of forgetfulness," have an equally insidious effect on us. These veils block our connection to our hearts, shroud us from the truth and "make us forget" that everything we need is actually already inside us. If we can just tap into our Divine wisdom, our temptations will fade into insignificance.

The "Veils of Forgetfulness"

Our society does all it can to avoid being uncomfortable. Look around: everything is designed to buffer discomfort. Take this pill. Don't say that. Don't rock the boat. Don't cry. It doesn't really hurt that much. And so on. We are conditioned to stay away from all feelings of discomfort, specifically emotional discomfort, rather than encouraged to stay with the experience and examine such feelings in order to see what we might be able to learn from them. As a result, we have not only learned to negate our own feelings but the connection with our body's innate wisdom to heal and balance itself.

Quite simply, we have lost touch with our emotional intelligence—we have lost connection with how we really feel. And in the process, we have forgotten our heart's wisdom. The more disconnected we are from feeling, the more we become numb and unresponsive to what's really important. If you are not connected to your heart, you have no way of navigating the world. You've lost connection to your soul's inner guidance system—your "soul's GPS" is offline!

These "veils of forgetfulness" are actually illusions, although they feel very real at the time. I call them "veils of forgetfulness" because they distort our perception of what is real and true for us, and derail our ability to navigate into the "remembrance" of our Heart's Wisdom.

The veils are formed when painful experiences occur in our lives. Loneliness, addiction(s), depression, fatigue, boredom, overstimulation and even death are the primary conditions that we tend to push away because of their associated discomfort. They "cause" us to experience a painful contraction in our heart, preventing us from seeing the Light that is coming through them. When this happens, we (unconsciously) create an avoidance pattern, a veil of forgetfulness. Instead of acknowledging the feeling and going within to see what might be at the root of it, we recoil in our forgetfulness and numb the pain with "something." We take the long way around, which of course never actually gets us there. But, when our focus is on integrating and growing from every experience, when we breathe deeply, and rest our attention in, and engage our hearts, we can dissolve these veils, get to the heart of the matter and become aware of the truth that lies within.

The real voyage of discovery consists not in seeking
new landscapes, but in having new eyes.
— *MARCEL PROUST*

Addiction

Addiction is one of the most concealing veils. It can be anything that we use or do that distracts us from feeling the emotional pain and discomfort and opening deeper to what lies within ourselves. Addiction starts when we attach a belief to something that fills an inner desire, and then we gradually come to rely on whatever "it" is—drugs, alcohol, sex, work, friends, shopping, sugar and so on—to feel okay. Before we know it we are hooked. Once the mind makes an association with the addiction as the object of our fulfillment, rather than finding that fulfillment from within, your connection to your heart becomes disengaged.

In actuality, you can never be fulfilled by that thing. You will only be fulfilled from within your deepest connection to yourself, your soul, and the wisdom of your heart.

When we are craving a certain feeling that we have attached to the object of our addiction, and are attempting to "scratch that itch" by indulging in the behavior to which we have become addicted, we can only ever find temporary satisfaction—because in reality nothing has actually changed. No matter how many times we feed it, that craving will never be truly satisfied. In no time at all, it will be back, and it will continue to control us, yearning for fulfillment, until we have met it at the Source and tasted the nectar of our "authentic self."

For if there is one habit or addiction we should endeavor to cultivate, this is it! One taste of that sublime connection to our authentic self is all it takes for us to become well and truly hooked. There is nothing like it. Once experienced, nothing else comes close, for the authentic self is the *only* source of true nourishment and personal fulfillment. All else pales in comparison. This is what you have been searching for; *this*, not your former addiction, is the "splinter in your mind" that has secretly been driving you "mad"... all the time!

One of the byproducts of addiction and the false sense of fulfillment that comes from the circle of craving is depression. Depression is also another veil. Its true nature might surprise you once we "unveil" this dark shadow that seems to have imprisoned so many people.

To understand the disharmony of human depression, it's important to understand its relationship to the earth (yes, there really is a relationship between the earth and depression!). Like all other living organisms, the earth is energetic in its essence. A distinguishing characteristic of energy is that it pulsates, and it has an undulating rhythm, just like the heart.

With training and practice, you can become aware of the dynamics of energy. Its pulse is always present and can be accessed as a powerful tool to reharmonize the body. As the primary pulse undulates, it rises into a peak and then descends into a valley. Each part of the cycle has a specific quality that you can tune into and use to assist your creative process and spiritual growth. The ebbs and flows of this and every cycle help us orient to a more natural and harmonious way of living.

The primary pulse has recognizable characteristics. During the "peak" phase, there is a rising feeling of inspiration; the "post-peak" phase, by contrast, feels like an afterglow, and there is a sense of sliding downhill into the "valley." The "valley" is, in fact, a return to stillness, or what Buddhists call formlessness; in fact, it is a deep drop inward into the stillness that lies at the center of our being, also known as the stillpoint. This drop is commonly mistaken for depression. But the truth is that it is here in the valley—in the void, the stillness—that the manifesting creativity is miraculously birthed.

Each aspect of the cycle must be nurtured in order to experience balance and optimal health. In our culture, most people are addicted to "peak" experiences and push the limits of their capacity, forcing themselves out of balance. Then, when they inevitably hit the "valley," they reach for the filler, that addictive "something" that will bring them back up to the peak, where they will (or so they believe) once again experience that sense of completeness that fuels their craving. But remember: a pendulum swings both ways. What goes up will come down—and sometimes it is not so pretty!

When we are addicted to the "peak," we work really hard to stay there because swinging back to the stillness of the center would mean having to be still with ourselves—with who we truly are. This is a scary thing when our whole lives have been orchestrated by our minds to be "outer-world focused," cut off from connection to our "inner world" and our hearts. Many people resist their own nature; they resist being completely themselves. This, of course, continuously keeps them out of balance. Then they wonder why they develop dis-ease, depression, addictions and imbalances in their body and in their lives.

Fatigue

Another Veil of Forgetfulness is fatigue, which is directly related to depression. Fatigue is a symptom that comes from a misinterpretation of being in the "Valley." The body needing to rest is one thing, but fatigue is quite another. When the body is burdened by limiting beliefs, over-stimulation, addiction and not being connected to the heart, the energy gets rerouted on an inefficient circuit; it wears on the body and makes it work harder than it should.

Our bodies are designed to maintain homeostasis—balance. Sleep is essential to health. During the sleep cycle, the REM (lighter Rapid Eye Movement sleep related to dreaming) and non-REM phases (delta, or slow-wave deep-sleep phase when body repairs take place) are designed to balance each other out. This is why people who do not fall into a deep enough sleep to experience the non-REM phase of the sleep cycle often feel tired, disoriented and sluggish in the morning; they are not well rested and, therefore, are "unbalanced."

In the same way, the "peaks" and "valleys" of our waking life need to balance each other out, too. Our bodies are in constant stress mode because we never take the time to relax consciously during the day. Conscious relaxation involves an entirely different set of skills and serves a purpose that sleep does not. By requiring us to remain in the present moment and simply bring mindful attention to what is going on in our bodies without judgment or trying to change anything, conscious relaxation starts to alter the neurological pathways in our brain. The more we practice mindfulness, the more readily we are able to tap into the Relaxation Response and move away from habitual fight-or-flight stress responses in our body that keep us on edge.

The problem is that many of us are so cut off from our feelings, and the messages that our bodies are sending us, we often don't even recognize when we have moved beyond the borders of mere tiredness and are in danger of entering the minefield of fatigue.

Here are some typical ways in which fatigue can affect us:

1. We start thinking too much! Thoughts go round and round in our head, rarely finding resolution. This draws too much energy into the head, leaving us feeling "off balance."

2. We develop poor eating habits: overeating, undereating, eating foods that are hard to digest or craving foods that never quite satisfy us.

3. We stuff down and ignore our emotional issues because we don't have the energy or fortitude to deal with them.

4. We can't sleep at night. Or if we do, we don't sleep very soundly. We're easily disturbed and find ourselves waking up every few hours. Consequently, we wake up tired, irritable and cranky, and end up dragging ourselves through the day.

5. We make excuses to stop exercising. This unwittingly creates a vicious cycle: the less aerobic exercise we get, the less oxygen we have to fuel our mind and body, the more fatigued and depressed we feel.

6. We become dehydrated. The more fatigued we are, the more prone we become to seeking an energy boost through instant pick-me-up sources like sugar, caffeine, sodas and other unhealthy foods and drinks, all of which can have a deleterious effect on the body's fluid balance.

7. We mismanage stress. When we are fatigued, it is harder to manage stress. And mismanaged stress creates more fatigue because the body is engaged in a constant holding pattern of tension.

Boredom

Another veil is boredom. If we are bored then we are not paying attention. We live in an infinite Universe, with infinite possibilities and opportunities on every level of consciousness. If you are bored, you are preoccupied with some limited perception of life. On some level, you have chosen to disengage from the wisdom of your heart that would otherwise be inspiring you, driving you forward, tempting and titillating you with passions and purpose.

I know this may sound harsh, but this is one of the golden fruits of this book. Life is ripe and bursting with—well, life! Dig in and join in the greatest party ever!

Okay, back to the veils. This is also true with the opposite of boredom: overstimulation. Being overstimulated is yet another effect of not engaging the heart, an inability to process all the multisensory and multidimensional information coming at you. You are absorbing everything, but your nervous system can't handle all of the stimuli and your body begins (in some cases quite literally) to freak out! When the body shuts down, the stimuli backs up within it, creating pressure, just like a pressure cooker.

As the pressure builds up inside you, you become increasingly anxious, sometimes to the point of panic. The trapped energy doesn't have an out. It is not circulating. From here, any number of things can happen, usually involving your mind hooking onto something external to make it feel better, which can be the seed of an addiction or the maintenance of one.

Why is this happening? The body becomes programmed through its conditioning to manage the day-to-day affairs of your life. You become "wired" in a certain manner to manage the energy to which you are accustomed. But as you grow and life changes, and especially as you find yourself subjected to the onslaught of a "consumerist regime," the system can become overloaded. Instead of taking steps to manage the overload, most people numb out, which is a strategy that provides temporary relief at best. Boredom and overstimulation lead us into the same numb, detached space, where we miss out on all the action, adventure and possibilities in the Universe.

When you understand what is happening when you get over-stimulated, it becomes self-evident what you need to do. You come to realize first and foremost that you need to let go, relax and let some steam out, by just allowing the energy to flow through you. You need to shut down the computer, television, radio, and other technologies, take time out for some conscious relaxation and slide into the "valley" to restore balance to your life. All of the behaviors outlined above will disengage your heart; they will send you off on a wild goose chase, in search of "things" that can never bring you the peace, juice and joy you desire! Anytime you notice yourself participating in them, all you have to do is take time out to engage your heart. The exercise at the end of this chapter will help free you. It only takes a moment to engage your heart!

The Veil of Death

There's another "veil" that's slightly different from the others, which often trips a lot of people up. This is the veil of Death.

When I was four years old, I used to enjoy watching *Sesame Street* on PBS. One day, another program came on straight afterward that captured my attention—in the worst possible way. The program was about death, and somehow, as I sat riveted to the television screen, I absorbed the message that I was going to die.

That was a little too much for my four-year-old mind to handle! The thought terrified me so much that I immediately erupted into tears and rushed into the kitchen, screaming to my mother, "I don't want to die! I don't want to die!" This traumatic event, which ultimately took root as a profound fear of death, stayed with me throughout most of my childhood and on into my adult life.

As it happens, it was this deeply irrational fear surrounding death, that I now realize first prompted me to engage in a deep exploration of life, in order to discover what was most important and real. Of course, this research could never have been complete until I forced myself also to take an honest, eyes-wide-open look at death. In the process, I came to realize that death is one of the most commonly avoided yet simultaneously painful experiences of our human existence. And as I gradually learned to resolve my own fear and pain around death, I also discovered a deeply profound and transformative process for quickly healing the immobilizing effects of grief, fear and loss. This transformative process has become an integral part of the Heart Wisdom process that you are now exploring within this book.

As my dear friend and colleague, Ian McKelvie, who is a Change Specialist and CEO of BECAUZ! once reminded me during a conversation we were having about the importance of exploring death: "If you can't be with death, you can't be fully present to life."

In Western culture, death is something we either "get over" or "get through." Death—understandably—causes us much discomfort, distress and pain, but since it is not a behavior, I can imagine that comparing it to the other veils here may seem rather strange. However, when we live from our fully engaged hearts, and are fully in touch with our "inner world" and our true selves, we know that death is not something to "get through" or "get over." Rather, it is something we simply need to *be* with.

Being with death allows our natural self-healing mechanism to support the opportunity that death affords. By opportunity, I mean that just like heartbreak, death is an opportunity to open more fully to the source of life, see the truth about what death really is and allow a new relationship to form. Remember, the body knows what to do. We do not have to figure it out. Shifting the paradigm on how we relate to death is the single most potent way to liberate a joyful and loving life!

As we heal our relationship with death, we come to see that mourning/grieving is an essential and truly rich experience of life. It is about taking the time to allow the natural healing and transformative process. Really, it is about engaging the heart. But most people try to cut this short. They put their minds on other things, instead of letting their hearts take over. They go back to work—get back to normal, or create as many "peaks" of activity and as few "valleys" of stillness as possible. This actually ends up achieving just the opposite of what was intended; it draws out the process because we never actually deal with the real issues at hand.

According to grief expert Aurora Winter, it typically takes between five and eight years to recover from a heartbreaking loss. When you grieve fully, allowing sufficient time for things to come up at their own pace and to process them with effective support, you create the perfect conditions to truly heal and allow something new to be born. In this way, you'll find that grieving isn't a long drawn out process of suffering and stagnation of life but a doorway to extraordinary peace and liberation.

I am going to share a truth that I have discovered about death and loss. Some of you may not be ready for this truth; yet, having helped many clients unravel and resolve their conflicting feelings and emotions around the death of a loved one or loss of a love, I have come to believe that what I am about to share could very well set you free on a whole new level.

We have been trained by society to treat death in a very somber way. Society conditions us to believe that if we truly loved someone, then there's something wrong with us if we don't demonstrate this with a prolonged display of grieving.

We are expected to feel grief and sadness for a very long time. If we laugh and enjoy ourselves, or if we go out and actually have fun when we are supposed to be filled with grief over our loss, people tend to assume that we didn't really care about our loved one. And so we feel guilty when we have those "feel-good" moments because society says we are supposed to feel bad. All of these heavy emotions of pain, misery and guilt cause us to contract our hearts and shut down.

The truth is that love never dies. The love that we once experienced is always available to us, because love *always* exists, regardless of whether we are separated from a loved one because of death, or for some other reason. Even if our partner were to leave us and run off with our best friend, the love we shared with them will still exist. It is we who close ourselves off from it through the contraction we experience *in reaction* to our loss.

Through the veil of death, we focus so much on pain, loss, guilt, depression, loneliness and similar feelings that we constrict and close down. What we have been taught by society is the right thing to do when we lose someone is actually the very worst thing for us.

The process doesn't have to be the way society has decreed. It is possible for us to let go of the feelings of grief and pain and replace them with the heart-opening warmth, expansion and love that allows us to enjoy the best memories of all the most wonderful times with a loved one without the pain. By connecting with the love that is and was always there, we can lift the veil of forgetfulness and death. We will feel the love physically in our body, and as we open the connection to our heart, we will be connected on the deepest soul level with our loved one—wherever they are. This inner work is rooted in the wisdom that "the truth will set you free."

Pulsing with Gratitude

Living in gratitude is one of the fastest ways to allow the energy of life to flow deliberately through your heart. It is about connecting with the source of life, the infinite energy and directing its vitality through your heart. When you do this, there is a tangible response within your body and, more specifically, within your heart. When the energy enters your heart and you allow your heart to be soft and open, it is like a flower releasing its sweetest fragrance. With practice you can access this "ability"—the ability to connect with and generate love and gratitude at will. Also realize that gratitude *is* love. When you feel gratitude, you are loving someone for something they did, or simply for who they are. Expressing gratitude is another form of sharing love.

Think of gratitude as a verb. It is love in action. Living in gratitude is a proactive step in creating your quality of life. It is not just about the space you are coming from; it is about gaining a sense of mastery in how you choose to show up in the world. Living in gratitude will give you a conscious connection to the Divine source, allowing you to approach the abundance of life and experience the generosity of creation as a daily practice and meditation. Whereas in the past looking on the bright side might have been a stretch, when you live in gratitude you live each and every day in a state of appreciation.

And here's the juice: Living in gratitude is rooted in the understanding that life itself is the supreme gift, as well as the most sublime gift of all. Everything else is simply a bonus. To allow yourself to realize this opens up infinite doors to loving opportunities and experiences. Allow yourself to see the mystery of life! At first it can be confounding to the mind and overwhelming to senses. But as you relax into it and soften you heart, you come to realize that life is just a pure gift that was given to you from nothing that you have done. Life asks nothing of you; it is a living demonstration of unconditional generosity... or love!

In your realization of this immense truth and truly connecting with it, you'll experience an overwhelming feeling of gratitude... and humbleness. Cultivate softness within your heart on a daily basis. Practice self-love—loving and comforting yourself and your heart as you would your own small child. Living in gratitude requires that you not only maintain a conscious connection with your heart, but also visualize your energy flowing through your heart as a means to generate love. Remember gratitude is love in action. As you begin to cultivate this "skill," you will realize that you can consciously generate gratitude and also regulate how much love you choose to feel in a given a moment.

When you begin to live your whole life in gratitude, you'll suddenly notice that you are in a place of spiritual power. The more you feel humbled and thankful for all the gifts of life, the more gifts seem to flow naturally to you. (At the end of this chapter, I have included a simple technique that will enable you to experience this place of spiritual power.)

Mastering Forgiveness

Mastering forgiveness is the second most powerful and effective way of engaging the heart, and overcoming the "veils" we've been discussing in this chapter. Forgiveness is about letting go. It is about *consciously choosing* to not hold on to an experience or person that is no longer serving your empowerment and/ or the ability to experience the fullness of love, life and joy! Holding onto hurt, pain and resentment is poison to your body and mind. If you become fluid in your ability to let go and restore peace and balance to your body, then you can experience joy, open to your heart and heal the wounds of the past.

In the past, when someone "did something" to you and you held on to it and/or didn't forgive, a contraction formed, you pulled back your love and closed off the heart. Your choice was to blame the other person, to not give love, but to withhold it. This is the opposite of forgiveness. Holding back love shuts the heart down. There can be no engagement of the heart, nor love of the Divine, when you are choosing to hold someone else responsible and choosing not to forgive. This, however, says something about your worthiness in the arena of love. That she or he left is not the issue. That he or she "did something" so unforgivable is not the issue. The issue is *what you have made this mean.*

If you are dependent on another person for your happiness, and he or she leaves you, then of course it is painful and indeed oftentimes devastating! But if you realize, or are open to, the possibility that the source of your happiness doesn't come from another, then, in essence, it won't matter if he or she is there or not. You won't need to close your heart because the person is no longer there to love. You will *be* love no matter what. You will continue to be loving, both to yourself and to others.

This was brought home to me by my friend Sandy, when she told me about "the best and most rewarding relationship" she had ever had. Sandy had known going into the relationship that the odds were stacked against it lasting. Johnny was twenty years younger than her, and while Sandy had had her reservations about "being a cliché," as she put it, she finally decided to follow her heart (and not her head), go with the flow, and just enjoy the moment. She never imagined that their "moment" would last for five years. When the time came for her and Johnny to part, though not without some pain on both sides, it nonetheless happened gracefully and lovingly. It wasn't the age gap that parted them, rather, it was their careers—Sandy was heading in one direction, while Johnny was heading in another, but both were determined to remain friends.

All was fine for several months. While Sandy missed Johnny, they stayed in regular contact and she was happy with her life. However, several months later, when Johnny and she were talking on the phone one day, he casually confided that he was starting a new relationship with a woman he had recently met. "That was when the truth of the situation finally sank in," she said. She and Johnny would never be together in the same way again.

The knowledge hurt. The emotions crowded in—hurt, abandonment, jealousy, resentment, regret and loss—Sandy sat with them all and allowed them to surface one after the other. She shed a tear or two, sighed over what might have been, and then, because she was essentially connected to her heart, she deliberately allowed her memory to take her back over all the little moments, incidents and experiences with Johnny that had confirmed for her how much she had gained from the relationship, and how very much she had been loved.

"That was the moment," Sandy confided to me, "when I realized that if you really love someone, that love can never die. No matter what happens, love always is. All we have to do is stay open to that knowledge, to that reality, and allow love to *be*. Several years later, Sandy and Johnny are still the very closest of friends. Anyone who sees them together instantly knows how much genuine love, affection and admiration they still—and will always—have for one another. By not demanding that their love for one another should look or be expressed in any specific way, but rather should just be allowed to be, they have managed to transform their former passion into a love of the highest and noblest order—the truly unconditional love that is known as agape!

This kind of behavior requires a core shift, the engagement of the heart and a willingness to stay wide open to love. Sandy could have chosen to respond to Johnny's new relationship in a multitude of "contracting" ways. Instead, she chose to feel her sadness and regret, and then simply let them go—no blame, no stories, no regret. The result is a beautiful, loving friendship that she and Johnny will undoubtedly share for the rest of their lives.

For most people however, the paradigm of relationship is much different than what Sandy and Johnny experienced. Many are entwined in the belief that the other person "completes" them. Thus if our lover is not there, we cannot possibly be happy. This is the core of codependence: we give away our power and become dependent upon another for our happiness.

But no one can *make* us feel happy. We are the only ones who can be responsible for our feelings and our reactions, and thus our happiness. The more conscious and open we are, the less prone to reaction we are. When we are unconscious, what someone says or does can "trigger" a reaction within us. The resulting friction then causes something to come up to the surface. If we are not conscious of what is happening, we will react as if the other person is *doing* something *to* us, when in fact it is *we* who are doing the *doing*.

It's important to remember that the other person can have stuff, too, but the goal here is to liberate ourselves. True liberation starts with taking responsibility for our own actions (and reactions), and instead of laying the blame elsewhere, choosing to look at what, where, when and how we can forgive. Being connected to our heart enables us to have an awareness of such things, to remain neutral and not be prisoner to an emotional charge. As *New York Times* bestselling author Debbie Ford, creator of *The Shadow Process,* says, "If nothing comes up it is just information; if you get triggered, if there is a charge, then it's your stuff."

HEART WISDOM KEY NUMBER SIX

Finding Forgiveness

Read through this exercise before you give it a try or simply go to the Heart Wisdom Web site (*www.heartwisdom.com*) and download the free MP3 recording.

1. Begin with a few minutes of deep breathing.

2. Practice the breathing exercises you have learned in this book.

3. Place your hands on your heart, ask your inner self, "Who, in my life, am I still feeling resentment toward over something they may have said or did, or neglected to say or do?"

4. Pause and make a list of all the people and the experiences that come to mind.

5. One by one rest your attention on each person/experience.

6. Allow all the feelings, emotions, thoughts and memories to surface.

7. Allow each thought, feeling, emotion and memory to pass through your "field of perception" like a cloud in the sky—like watching the credits roll on a movie screen.

8. Give yourself permission to feel every emotion and experience as deeply and fully as possible.

9. Any time you notice yourself getting caught up in a particular thought or feeling, simply bring your attention gently back to your heart, take a few deep breaths and then resume your allowing.

10. Do this exercise for at least 10 minutes.

11. When you feel complete, write in your journal about your experience. Repeat as necessary.

12. For a deeper experience, do this exercise 10 minutes every day for one week straight.

HEART WISDOM KEY NUMBER SEVEN

Connecting with Love
You Thought You Had Lost

Here is an exercise to help you connect with the love you shared with someone whose loss you are still grieving. It can be someone who has passed on or an ex-lover or partner or spouse who you didn't want to lose. The purpose of this exercise is to revitalize all the love, laughter and joy you shared with them, and to connect with their living soul right here in the now. Remember that you can go to the Heart Wisdom Web site (*www.heartwisdom.com*) and download the free MP3 recording.

1. Begin with a few minutes of deep conscious breathing to settle your energy, relax your body and bring your attention present.

2. Mentally set your intention to connect with that particular person on a soul level, and give yourself 100 percent permission to receive the greatest gifts that become available for you during this experience. (Note: It's a choice to let it work for you. Give yourself the best opportunity to receive benefit by playing full on!)

3. Next bring your attention to rest in your heart. If it helps to physically connect with your heart, bring your hands to rest on your chest.

4. Continue breathing and begin thinking of a time when you were with this person when their truest and most authentic self was shining through.

5. As you begin to connect, let your heart feel all the feelings, emotions and sensations that arise. (Note: conjuring a memory creates a portal/access point for you to connect in present time with them. As you begin to feel a connection, allow the memory to fade and allow whatever is surfacing to rise naturally.)

6. Give yourself permission to feel the full essence and presence of their soul for your greatest peace and well-being.

7. Allow whatever is happening. If there are thoughts, allow the thoughts. If there are images, allow the images. If there are memories, allow the memories. Do the same with all emotions and feelings and sensations that you experience. Whatever is happening is perfect for this moment.

8. Spend as much time on this as you feel comfortable. When you feel complete, take a few more deep, full breaths and bring your attention back to your body in this present moment.

9. When you are ready, write in your journal about your experience.

Journaling is powerful vehicle to integrate your experience. It brings the energetic and emotional experience into the physical world. Because journaling draws on a different part of the brain to write than it does to visualize and do inner work (process), it creates additional neural pathways (connections in the brain). In so doing, it grounds the experience in the body and allows you to derive maximum benefit from the exercise.

CHAPTER SEVEN

Integrating Heart Wisdom

This is your last chance. After this, there is no turning back. You take the blue pill—the story ends; you wake up in your bed and believe whatever you want to believe. You take the red pill—you stay in Wonderland and I show you how deep the rabbit hole goes.

— MORPHEUS, THE MATRIX

As you've probably gathered by now, one of my all-time favorite movies is *The Matrix*. What I love about this movie is that besides being wildly entertaining, this science-fiction story shines a spotlight on how many of us live a life of delusion. In the fictional universe of the film, living human bodies are held in pods to generate energy for the ruling machines while the humans' mental, emotional and spiritual lives are contained and controlled in an artificial world called *The Matrix*. We are told and understand ourselves to be free, but more often than not we wake up day after day to the treadmill of life. We're just going through the motions, unable to stop, but never really moving forward to live the life we came here to live and experience the fulfilling life that we know to be possible, and believe in our hearts to be true.

Dissolving the Delusions

Our conditioned reality is, as Morpheus calls it, "a prison for our mind." Yet, as the film also suggests, there is hope. Outside *The Matrix* and outside our current perception of reality is another world where

> **HEART FACT**
>
> If you squeeze a tennis ball you are using about the same amount of force it takes your heart to pump blood to your body. The heart muscles work twice as hard, non-stop, as your leg muscles do when you are running as fast as you can.

our true selves blossom freely and contribute toward the creation of a new and liberated world. But in order to reach this place, we must "unplug" from our own living "matrix," and break through to this new world by piercing the veil of our own delusion.

This is something we cannot do without the practice of Heart Wisdom. As one of my teachers would say, "We don't realize the condition in which we find ourselves." We don't always notice how severed we feel from the Divine. We don't see how much we are living our lives as victims, resigned to accept the brutal mistreatment of the earth and so many of its inhabitants.

We may have even reached the place where we think this is normal. In this resignation, we've become blind to the immense power that we hold inside us, a power that, if harnessed properly and consciously, can literally change our lives and the world around us. We don't understand what is possible and available— what is happening right here right, now under our very noses.

Unless we integrate the practice of Heart Wisdom, we cannot unite with the intelligence that helps dissolve our delusions. Conversely, when we can connect with where we are, how we are living, and what we are contributing to the world, the Heart Wisdom practice provides a clear and focused approach to opening us up to a deeper understanding of ourselves, and our relationship to the Universe. It allows us to pierce the veils that obscure our vision of Divine reality. It incinerates the distortions of perception and the experience of the very nature of reality itself and allows the living Light of God to shred all illusion and delusion.

With each breakthrough that we experience and integrate into our daily life, the veils become thinner and eventually fall away, and so does the perception of who we are. We are stripped of our attachment to identity and are opened up to something greater. There is no longer a "me"—the "I" that is experiencing things dissolves and merges with the Divine, part of a greater spiritual being, albeit one who is having a human experience for a time. After experiencing this reality, it no longer makes sense to allow ourselves to feel weighted down and constricted by mundane disappointments or self-criticisms. Now we are free to create our lives differently.

This journey from the duality of everyday perception to the unified consciousness that lies beneath it is both surprising and awe-inspiring—a thoroughly enjoyable, comfortable place that no words can adequately describe. Here we are simply humble witnesses to something greater than ourselves, surrounded by the energy of the Light of the Divine. It is clear now that in order to be free we must no longer limit ourselves; we must join our own personal light to this "Light that casts no shadows" and allow it to radiate into the world around us.

Indeed, once we have had such an experience of what it means to be one with the Divine Light, it is no longer possible to turn away and withhold the gifts we have to offer the world. The brilliant and impassioned Andrew Harvey, author of *The Hope: A Guide to Sacred Activism* and a dear friend of mine, puts it this way: "When you have an authentic connection with the Divine, you are not motivated to *get* more; you are unabashedly inspired to *give* more!"

As you learn to develop your own Heart Wisdom practice, you will go deeper and deeper, creating sparks that ignite breakthroughs in all shapes and sizes, depths and textures. In the midst of a breakthrough, you will find that "it"—the constriction, the barrier, that thing that has been holding you back—isn't about what you thought it was about.

Where your breakthrough takes you will no doubt surprise you, but the more you experience this, the more familiar the terrain of your "inner world" will become. You will be dissolving and unwinding the contractions of the heart, body, mind and soul, moving beyond the trauma of unresolved emotions and negative beliefs and healing your deep emotional wounds. Your breakthroughs will uncover your deep wisdom, liberate your love, and transform the very nature of how you experience life.

The "Aha!" Moment

The word "breakthrough" can be misleadingly simple. It implies that your work is done—that you've broken through the barrier that has been holding you back and have come out the other side. All too often, the breakthrough *is* the end of the story. In fact, if you think back on your life, I would bet you could pinpoint a time when you experienced a breakthrough but no substantial change in your life appeared as a result. You felt the "Aha!" moment and then a day, a week or a month later you found yourself back where you were before.

The breakthrough is not the end; it is merely the beginning. We see this in *The Matrix* when Neo wakes up to find he has been freed from the Matrix, and asks Morpheus, "Why do my eyes hurt?" Morpheus responds, "You've never used them before."

Neo believed he was using his real eyes when he was inside the Matrix, but now that his delusion has dissolved and shifted to The Truth, the old way of seeing no longer serves him. He cannot go back to the old way, and so he must move forward, integrating this new knowledge and way of viewing the world into a new way of living. It is then that he finds his mission—his vehicle for sharing his gifts—and his daily existence blossoms, from a dead-end job and secret life as a computer hacker to an integrated life filled with purpose, meaning, energy and passion!

> **HEART FACT**
>
> "Did you know that the electrical impulses of your heart beats are registered by the brains of other people around you?"

It is, of course, important to let go of the form or expectation of what your breakthrough (and what happens after it) will look like. Whenever I facilitate relationship workshops with couples that are either having problems, or believe their relationship could be more fulfilling, I begin with the statement: "I am not committed to you staying together."

This may come as a surprise and can be downright scary to those who've experienced traditional couples counseling. In these workshops I am absolutely committed to guiding people in opening themselves up to the greatest possible love of their lives. I support each of them individually in their deepest truth. There, they can see the reality of their connection—how they connect, if they do connect.

In some cases, couples find they aren't connecting at all or that they have come together out of dysfunction. The only questions that matter are these: Is their current way of relating to each other serving their greatest loving? Or are they interfering in each other's process of creating that greatest love? This is not about being in a relationship or hanging in there together. And most of all, it is not about relying on another person to fulfill you. It is about breaking through whatever is holding you back from that greatest love, and that greatest fulfillment, and going where that leads you. The hitch is that once the breakthrough happens, you've got to be able to move with it.

While many books and programs are designed to support you in breaking through in a specific area of your life, they take the breakthrough as an endpoint. This chapter, though, is concerned with helping you go beyond the initial moment of the "Aha!" to integrate that understanding into your everyday life.

Like Neo, I want you to live an integrated life filled with purpose, meaning, energy and passion!

In reality, much of what we experience as a breakthrough ends up being just a glimpse of something beyond ourselves and our present way of living. We wake up to where we really are, and who we really are. We understand in a heartbeat that we are whole beings—body and spirit, inner and outer, human and Divine are one—and that there is a living source of life mysteriously and miraculously radiating the astonishing light of God, and wow! does it change the way we see and experience the world... at least for a moment!

It is an amazing moment and one that can throw open every door and pathway of possibility, transforming fear to love, chaos to calm and confusion to clarity! However, if we don't consciously *integrate* the new vision into our daily lives, then we have not really *broken* through anything, but have only *peeped* through a hole in the wall that has been blocking us from our wholeness and fulfillment.

The vision we have been given of something greater is a gift. However, it's what we do with it that shapes and sculpts the very fabric of our lives. Will you lapse back into old negative beliefs or emotional patterning? Or will you bring the breakthrough, the healing, the love, the peace and the Light of God back into the human experience? Are you willing to take that courageous step and do things differently?

Blue pill or red? You choose.

In *The Matrix*, the truth-seeing Oracle leads Neo to believe that he is not the "One," the savior that the liberated humans have been waiting for to rid the world of the Matrix and free the humans from the machines' rule. Neo acts on the information he is "given," but later he finds out that the information is wrong. Even so, the outcome of his actions is positive—he saves Morpheus' life.

Morpheus explains to Neo that the Oracle told him what he needed to hear. In other words, there was a deeper wisdom being communicated here. Guidance from our intuitive intelligence is not necessarily truth to be taken literally. It is a more sublime intelligence that prompts us to take the necessary action that would have eluded us had we taken it as literal truth.

Morpheus says, "Neo, sooner or later you're going to realize, just as I did, that there's a difference between knowing the path and walking the path." Walking the path/living the path is about being present to a deeper intelligence and responding to a deeper calling. Neo had to be present to his "gut instinct" and trust his flow, to act without getting caught up in semantics, entangled in expectations, or distracted by "the story."

Conscious Integration

The "Aha!" moment is often the first level of a breakthrough. It is a glimpse into something beyond your normal perception where you achieve a new awareness. This is an awakening from the human condition. You become aware of a depth and richness of your inner world and the possibilities that open up when you live from the heart instead of your head. You connect or tap into something Divine within and beyond yourself.

The "Aha!" moment doesn't have to be dramatic or earth shattering, it can be as simple and straightforward as it was for Neo, when he simply realized what it was that he needed to do. It can happen anywhere, when you are doing anything. Suddenly, like a shooting star, or slowly, like a sunrise, your view of the world and your place in it shifts slightly. You become ultra-present to the moment, the magic of the world around and beyond you.

It may be during an evening walk in the woods, when you suddenly become aware that you are hearing all of the individual sounds around you. It may be an amazing meal you've prepared or been served, and you find yourself tasting the flavorful dimensions of every bite. You have a glimpse, albeit ever so slight, of what is possible in the world and in your life. It is sensory—a conscious tapping-in to a living intelligence that alters how you think, feel, and relate to and in the world.

The "Aha!" moment begins the work of clearing out stuck energy from past experiences and unkinking the hose connecting us to our true self and our Heart Wisdom. Much of the stuck energy that we are clearing out is the result of what we explored in Chapter Five: negative beliefs and trapped emotions from difficult experiences, like the death of a close friend or family member, betrayal or heartbreak. It is important to remember that these events, when buried or unprocessed, become the stuck energy that can block our connection to our bodies, inner worlds, our hearts and its wisdom.

If your breakthrough stops here with the "Aha!" you have indeed received a precious gift. You've moved some energy and your perception will have shifted.

But basically you've just rearranged the furniture in the house. It looks a little different, it might even feel different, but it's all aesthetic. Very soon the dust will settle again, the spiders will begin spinning their webs and, one day, you will look up from your treadmill and realize that life is just the same.

When you are willing and able to consciously integrate your breakthrough, stay open, and allow this energy to keep moving, you maintain your connection to your Heart Wisdom and the flow of the Universe; as a consequence, all aspects of your life begin to blossom in a whole new way. Then you will have a quantum shift in how you show up and experience life. You may have heard the saying that 80 percent of life is just showing up. Well, I would actually say that 100 percent of life is showing up! And showing up 100 percent is what affords you the great opportunity of being met and graced by the extraordinary generosity of the Infinite.

One client of mine, whom I'll call Jerry, had been struggling for about six months with his "breakthrough" because he was yet to integrate it into his life. He had done a lot of inner work and come to the realization that there was a yawning gap between the life he was living and the one he really wanted. But with that breakthrough came frustration that he had seen the truth but didn't know how to move toward it.

In one of our sessions together, Jerry had his "Aha!" moment when he realized that the barrier that was holding him back from the life he really wanted was the story he'd constructed. In truth, anything that is holding us back comes from our story—our unconscious or subconscious beliefs and interpretations of who we think we are and how we understand life and our relationships with others.

Jerry's story came up in a few different ways, but they could all be boiled down to a singular fear: his fear for personal survival. Jerry was a go-go-go kind of person, always pursuing more money, more achievement, more success, even more spiritual growth, and never feeling that there was enough time in his life to pack in all the "more-more-mores" that constantly drove him. It got so bad that upon waking up in the morning, Jerry's first conscious reaction was one of panic—his heart would begin racing like a rat on an exercise wheel.

Through the work we did together, he finally was able to recognize that his underlying belief was one of scarcity: if he didn't do more, he wouldn't have "enough," and if he didn't have "enough" he would never feel secure. With the recognition that this scarcity-based belief was the juice he was addicted to, Jerry also realized that the "juice" that fed him was the same "juice" that deluded him. "Aha!"

An epic wrestling match began with Jerry's "Aha!" He'd feel joyful and free until weeks, days, hours or minutes later. Then his "scarcity" story would raise its ugly head and overpower him again, causing a knot of self-doubt in the pit of his stomach. His only "weapon" was to stay in the moment, breathe deeply, welcome the story and open to the wisdom of his heart. That knot of self-doubt was Jerry's teacher. It said, "Hey, you're "missing" something—pay attention. There's a gift here for you!"

Jerry and I worked together to unwind the knot. Had Jerry been working on this own, he could easily have succumbed and let the "Aha!" moment end right there. But he wasn't alone. His wife was on the same path, and he also had me as his "storybuster." Whenever his scarcity stories showed up in our sessions, I would simply point them out and remind him that he had the choice to delete or dissolve the delusion.

As we continued our work, Jerry developed more and more of awareness around these stories, and the ways in which they held him back from what he really wanted in life. Using the Heart Wisdom practice, he became very adept at to navigating his inner world in order to free himself from his "stories." That's not to say that the move from that "Aha!" moment level to the next level of integration was easy or short for Jerry, but it was simple. It was not a matter of *doing* but of *allowing*, welcoming, breathing and sticking with it. This is essential to deepening the breakthrough, to integrating the "Aha!" and achieving the change you so deeply desire. It doesn't have to be a "peak" experience. With patience, the assistance of a "storybuster" and the grace of God, it can be gentle, simple and, most important of all, permanent.

So now let's look a little more closely at this concept of integration.

The word integration is typically defined as: an act or instance of combining into an integral whole. It originates, in part, from the word integrity, which means: the state of being whole, entire, or undiminished. Typically, the word "integrity" is also used to refer to your sense of honor: Do you follow through with the commitments you make? Can people count on you? Is your handshake worth anything?

In short, integrity is how much you stand behind your "word." In common usage, when you are out of integrity, you have broken your word. Thus, when someone accuses you of being out of integrity, it usually has a negative connotation. Your accuser thinks you are wrong for doing something that is not congruent with what you promised, or what you claim to be your values.

Integral Living

However, if we delve a little deeper into the meaning of "integrity," we find that it also relates to the essential or integral connection you have with yourself. Integrity here means wholeness, completeness. So being in integrity is being in a state of wholeness—experiencing an essential connection with the wholeness of your being. In this sense, being in integrity means being connected to and expressing the fullness of you, whereas being out of integrity means, coming from a place that is expressing anything less than that fullness.

You are out of integrity when you are not living in coherence with that inherent, fundamental and vital connection with the wholeness of life and your Heart Wisdom. When you realize that you are living out of integrity, it is not good or bad. Instead, it is an awesome opportunity to open more fully to your essential connection with your heart. When you are out of integrity, the person you are "hurting" the most is you; however, you are also doing a disservice to the world because you are not sharing your unique gifts, and your light is "diminished." Being in integrity allows your energy to flow in its greatest abundance and clarity through your body and your life. As a result, the greatest of all possibilities can be born. It opens you to unbounded creativity, prosperity, energy, joy, love and true fulfillment in your life.

When you consciously integrate an "Aha!" into your life, you feel the truth and opportunity of a new awareness; you feel and experience yourself as a spiritual being. You begin to be guided and to move from a deep place. You see that you can consciously choose your behavior. You choose to use the Heart Wisdom practice, to breathe deeply, drop into your heart, unwind your body and make your decisions and live your life from there. At this level you are making conscious choices to keep up the practice and see the world with your new eyes, dissolving delusions easily, without defaulting to past patterning.

Conscious integration can feel like a wrestling match, as with Jerry's struggle to stick with his breakthrough. It can be uncomfortable, frustrating, and even painful. It can also be graceful, flowing and instantaneous. Whether we recognize it or not—the choice is ours. Life is always seeking the path of least resistance—it is seeking its own liberation, although it doesn't always feel that way.

However the integration reveals itself, remember that what is at stake here is your life, and, if that isn't enough, consider what you can contribute to the world once you are free to share your gift. Remember that integration or living in integrity with your Heart Wisdom will bring your life to a whole new level. By dropping into the heart, connecting with the magic of life and remaining open, you will be integrating the inner (God) and outer (human) worlds—with integration you realize and embrace yourself as a spiritual being living a human life. That's powerful!

By opening to this heart wisdom and integrating that energy flow into every part of your life, you are grounding your being in your authentic place of power, in your wholeness and fullness, in the cosmic sweet spot of life. This is where the magic is. This is where miracles occur. The truth of the matter is that once we open to this exquisite love force and begin to experience the benefits of living from our heart, there is no going back.

Keep in mind, however, that being connected doesn't mean you won't have challenges to deal with. It just means you are better equipped to handle whatever comes down the pipeline of your life. How will you stay open in the midst of chaos? Will you default to old patterning, or stay open, alive with integrity, present in the moment and able to grow from every experience?

HEART WISDOM KEY NUMBER EIGHT

Integrating Heart Wisdom

Integration is vital to living a joyful and loving life. Integration is about grounding the cultivation of our Heart Wisdom in our physical world, which includes our bodies, the earth, our relationships, and our life's work.

A Zen teacher once said that we must "reinvest our inner cultivation." This means that what we have tapped into, healed and experienced in our inner-world exploration needs to be brought forth and grounded in the world in a meaningful way. There is no wrong way to do this. It just has to be meaningful for you. For example, this book is a reinvestment of my "inner cultivation." It is a culmination and synthesis of some of the most valuable truths I have experienced.

Please note that it does not have to be as grandiose as writing a book. It can be as simple as writing a poem, organizing a community cleanup, having that long overdue conversation with that certain someone, or even a simple apology to someone you have hurt. Again, it just has to be truly meaningful to you, inspired by your tapping into the wisdom of your heart. (Remember you can go to the Heart Wisdom Web site, *www. heartwisdom.com*, and download the free MP3 recording):

1. Take a few deep breaths and center your attention in your heart.

2. Recall an Aha! moment and/or breakthrough experience you have had in the process of doing this Heart Wisdom work.

3. Bring the memory of that moment into your heart.

4. Mentally ask yourself: "What would be the most beneficial reinvestment of this breakthrough back into my life?

5. Sit with the answer in your heart for at least five minutes, or until you really feel something significant bubble up from the depth of your Heart Wisdom.

6. Once you are clear, take out your journal and write down what it is and make a plan to execute it. Make sure to include all the steps you will need to take to complete the action. This will make it easy for you to follow through. If possible and, if applicable, write down the timeline to bring this to fruition.

DO IT!

CHAPTER EIGHT

Unification

We all share the wound of fragmentation. And we can all share
in the cure of unification. Healing is the unification of all our forces
—the powers of being, feeling, knowing, and seeing.

— *GABRIELLE ROTH*

Integration is the final key to mastering Heart Wisdom. When you reach this final phase, your thoughts and actions are all governed by the desire to keep this channel open. It affects everything—how you walk, speak, eat, think, move, even how you breathe. You ask yourself, does this action, decision, food, argument, empower and/or support my openness? This is the Great Practice—this is what enables you to stay open and expand your heart's capacity to experience love, life and unity with God and yourself!

Of course, there are plenty of "veils" and "delusions" that will appear and distract you from staying open. For as with any transformational experience, you will always come to a place, your edge, in which you will be "challenged"—not only by your ability to trust your inner intelligence, but also by the question of whether or not your spirit is guiding you in a beneficial direction. The secret to staying open through this is very simple: it lies in continuously practicing and applying the techniques for accessing your Heart Wisdom that you have learned in this book.

This is how you take the journey from the head *through* the heart. But this is not a quest in the traditional sense. The truth is that nobody ever actually reaches God… because God is already *here*. There is nowhere to go and nothing to reach for. For there *is* only HERE and NOW.

Infinite Possibilities

You really can connect to the space of infinite possibilities and create the life you want. When you experience yourself unhooked from your mental perceptions (your mind's beliefs, ideas, stories and interpretations), you realize that the way you choose to live in any given moment is only one of infinite possibilities that are available to you. In this awareness, you are free to create your life as you choose or are guided to choose—thus the question then becomes: "What do I choose?" or "What does God choose for me?"

Remember, you may have entered this transformational journey feeling limited in your choices, but once you have opened to a certain degree, you inevitably come face to face with the Infinite. Where you once felt limited with your choices, you now are overwhelmed with them; it is a powerful place to be and though it can be somewhat daunting, it is the very best kind of challenge to have. However, it does indeed require some delicacy and keen inner navigation skills to remain on the path. "Attaining" integration and unification means that you now have access to all of the resources of your own Heart Wisdom and, therefore, the means to handle anything that comes into your life.

You now enjoy a relationship of trust with yourself, the Universe and the world around you. You realize through experience that everything is connected and we are all interwoven in one dynamic and multidimensional orchestration of life. Feeling part of this relationship, you can now see how the Universe supports you because you feel yourself a part of it. You feel its benevolence and supportive nature and it becomes astonishingly obvious that it is a *supportive* Universe that simply is "conspiring to support you." You are no less supported than the soil that is nourished by the rain or the flower that is fed by the sun.

From here you have nothing to fear. You feel taken care of from within, and have the certainty that life always has "your best interest in mind." You receive what is being offered and move through life with a trust that is beyond words. You become a lover of what is, not what you *think* should be! In your heart connection, you realize that you don't need life or others to be any different than they already are. You have come to accept the flow of life and you rejoice in its unfolding. You see and feel yourself a part of it in the same way that you feel another person, or a tree, or the earth as part of your own body. You see it as it is, through the eyes of God, through the eyes of Love!

It is your heart that affords you the gift of seeing this truth of who you are. Your heart *is* the golden key to your kingdom, the crown jewel of your life! But this only becomes "self-evident" when your heart has broken open and has been healed in the purifying fires of "heart break-down to heart break-through." Or what author and spiritual teacher Andrew Harvey refers to as "crucifixion by love!"

In this rebirth, you are in a new relationship with life. You are linked into your Heart Wisdom and able to access your inner intelligence. You allow your intuition to guide you to the right choices and determine which of the infinite possibilities are appropriate for you. Your heart connection brings you into the present moment and enables you to respond instead of react.

For example, if someone cuts you off on the highway, are you responsible for his or her actions? Of course not; that is their responsibility. But you *are* responsible for your participation in it. What this means is that on a deeper level you showed up to be the recipient of that action. For example, let's take the case of the highway incident, which is something we are all familiar with. What if the person who cut you off was actually putting you out of harm's way? Or what if that incident was an opportunity for you to learn to not react and lose your temper over others' actions, and thereby master the bigger lesson of not allowing what another person says or does to control you or your sense of peace and well-being?

When viewed from a higher perspective we can see that this is very deep stuff inasmuch as it requires us to be equally responsible in our interactions with others, even when we are not the initiator of a difficult or awkward situation. And this is where the shift in consciousness has to occur. Einstein said, "You can't solve a problem with the same level of thinking that created it." When you are in your head, you will never understand how you contributed to someone else cutting you off. You must unhook your mind and transcend your intellect. Otherwise, your mind will tell you that the other person is a (fill in your favorite derogatory word or phrase), and look to blame that person for what just occurred.

One of the biggest lessons we all need to learn is that we can never know what is really happening, for there is always a higher perspective to consider. But when you are being in the moment and coming from your heart, you have the greatest vantage point to instinctively respond or intuitively make the best decisions. When you are unified with the Divine through your connection to your Heart Wisdom, you will not only find it much easier to make conscious choices that reflect a new and deeper understanding of yourself and the world around you but you also will find yourself responding from your heart in every situation.

Conscious Communication

An important part of integrating your Heart Wisdom into your everyday life is to make a shift in how you communicate with other people. In our mind-centered society, most people speak from their cluttered, spinning minds, so what comes out is cluttered and spinning. They speak with no awareness of their inner self, their soul or their heart, so their expression isn't very substantial. When you are open, you are clearer; there is a qualitative substance that is transmitted in the fluidity of your voice, and it becomes very obvious where you are coming from!

Either we are growing or dying, generating life or depleting life. So it is with our communications. Every time we open our mouths, what we choose to say has the opportunity to be life generating or life depleting, our chance to share love and life. With practice, our communications can become a means of loving service—a gift of nourishment with each word and utterance.

But remember: talking is only part of the communication experience; deep listening is also necessary. The value of truly hearing oneself and hearing another speak cannot be underestimated in any relationship. It is the seed of true intimacy and the foundation for lasting love. Strangely, "listening" is a skill that we are rarely taught growing up. Yet it *is* a skill that we would all do well to learn. I have watched many of my clients reverse seemingly impossible situations, after learning a few simple tools that I taught them. Just by learning deep listening, their lives have become fulfilled beyond their expectations, and strangely enough, they have learned to really hear themselves as well as those they care about.

The Number One Culprit in Communication Struggles

The majority of struggle in relationships comes from the core dynamic that arises when one person *thinks* he or she understands what the other is saying. In that assumption they forge forward in the conversation without really connecting. The result is two people talking *at* each other, rather than truly, deeply communicating. Have you ever noticed that when someone feels that they are not being heard, they start to talk louder, *thinking* that if they talk louder somehow they are going to be understood? The fundamental problem is not in the volume; it is in the *listening*.

One of the ways I support my clients in enhancing their listening skills, and in turn their communication and intimacy, is to have them reflect back what they *think* they heard the other person say.

You would be amazed how often this simple step reveals profound misunderstandings that would otherwise have slipped through the radar. The reason for this is two-fold: One is our lack of skill in listening—too often our minds are racing ahead, thinking about the response we wish to make, before we have even heard what is being said; the other is that not many people actually *say* what they really mean.

You may indeed reflect back accurately what the other has said, but it may not be what they meant. When people hear you reflect back what they said, it gives them a chance to refine their communication until the essence of what they really want to convey is spoken and heard. Then you can really *hear* one another, instead of escalating into further misunderstanding and, ultimately, complete frustration, which is where most relationships end up getting destroyed.

The simple tool of reflecting back what you have heard places more emphasis on connecting in true intimacy rather than on "getting your point across," or just "being right." In particular, it does wonders for your intimate relationship (hint: deep listening is the greatest aphrodisiac). More than anything else, deep listening demonstrates that what your partner says is important, and by listening you let him/her feel how much you value and cherish them.

Notice that hiding within the word communication is the word "commune," which is to come to a place of union, a common meeting place. Simple tools can set the ground that serves as that common meeting place for true communion to occur. For example, one of the most powerful and simplest tools (when you remember!) is to breathe while you speak. When you breathe while you speak, your attention naturally shifts from your head to your body. This allows energy to circulate, which nourishes and relaxes the body, and facilitates an easier engagement of the heart. Here is where two hearts can meet. And when two hearts meet, and two people truly connect in a common place, truly commune, it is nothing short of heaven.

Becoming Present

Achieving a union with the heart, spirit and self is about being present. This can be challenging in everyday life because there are so many distractions. But when you become adept at using the Heart Wisdom practice—getting out of your mind, bringing your attention inward, releasing your emotional blockages and engaging your heart—then you are free to be present, right here, right now.

"Peak" experiences often have the effect of pulling us away from the present. But even in such distracting, exciting or even traumatic moments, there is a chance to bring ourselves home to the present. When we have a powerful emotional experience, or when something feels traumatic, we are not "seeing" it with clear eyes/perception; we do not understand it as coming from a deep place within us. The point of our spiritual journey (and the opportunity at hand) is to "return home"—to connect with Source and experience the truth of who we are!

The only way to heal and change our life is to open to a deeper connection within us—to go inside, penetrate beneath the surface tensions and habits of the mind and emotions. We must "pierce the veil" of our contractedness and allow it to unwind and open us. The body already knows exactly what to do: return to the heart. All we have to do is follow.

Whenever a "peak" experience is not integrated, there is an unresolved energy residue from the experience. In most cases, our minds have made it mean something; therefore, there is a belief, a mental pattern/program that is "holding" the energy of the experience in place. And with that program alive in us, whenever we are looking to do something new that challenges that paradigm, our mind will automatically "defend its territory/livelihood."

The mind only knows what it knows, and it always acts to further survival and self-preservation. For a long time, the mind has been in control. But whatever it thinks it knows is already past, not present. This is crucial. The mind is coming from a place it knows: the past. But the present is wild and unbridled! Life is unfolding to its own rhythm, and what is unfolding is fresh and new. We have no idea what will happen next.

Right here, right now, just be in this moment, this present-time moment. See, hear, feel it unfold. There is nothing known about it. If your mind engages, it will contract the moment and try to interpret, give it meaning and simply take you out of the infinite extraordinariness that is unveiling itself before you. As Nick Nolte says in the movie, *The Peaceful Warrior*, "There are no ordinary moments." Remember: "If you aren't living in awe, you aren't paying attention."

I am truly inspired to do this work, and the reason is simple: over and over, I have witnessed the miracles it creates in my clients—amazing transformations, from suffering and misery to joyful living and loving. The shift that takes place in your inner foundation has an immediate and lasting effect on your behavior, thoughts and feelings. This is not so strange. There is no way that you cannot have a profound shift in your awareness when you are close to that level of Unification. I call it a "whole being breakthrough."

At first, signs of progress may not be so obvious, as they can emerge in so many different ways. But as you inch closer, everything in your life will start to reflect it: from your relationships and how you feel, to your body, mind and even your work. Your whole world is converging into this moment. Everywhere you turn, you will see signs of inevitability.

Then it begins to escalate, knocking a little more incessantly, gnawing at your attention, until the pressure/the force moves you into a sort of inner chaos. Nothing seems to makes sense, everything feels overwhelming; you cannot seem to make heads nor tails of anything—confusion, frustration, angst.

That's because there is a slippery slope effect at this level of breakthrough. The Ego, which is in charge of defending the status quo and staying in the past, will do everything in its power to neutralize your breakthrough. It will "try" to talk you out of it, intellectualize it, doubt it, poke holes in it and contain it—anything, in fact, to prevent it.

This is especially true if your breakthrough is about to move you out of your head, the Ego's palace, and into your heart. To integrate the breakthrough in a way that creates lasting change, you have to keep working until the Ego is exhausted and finally relents. The Ego is not bad. It is just doing exactly what it was programmed to do. The Ego's main focus is to defend what it is familiar with, what it knows, to create safety. The irony is that unification with your heart, self and the Divine is the only real safety you will ever know!

Whole Being Breakthrough

Do you remember my client Jerry and his "Aha!" moment that I related in Chapter Seven? Well, after many months of developing his practice of Heart Wisdom, Jerry, too, achieved Unification. In time, Jerry's "Aha!" of recognition—that his barrier was built out of his story—deepened into the awareness that there was a distance between the story and his true self. The story was not "him." It was this recognition and willingness to surrender his story that enabled Jerry's growth. As long as he kept up the fight, resisting it at every turn, Jerry's story held all the power. As soon as he breathed into it, took a good look at it, accepted it, even embraced it, the story relaxed its grip.

Jerry described his relationship with his "story" as being a bit like sibling rivalry: the story was the neglected little brother who invented all kinds of antics in order to get attention. Jerry only had to turn to this little brother and lavish him with the attention he craved and the wild child turned to a fluffy little kitten. Every part of us, including our stories, just wants to be acknowledged, loved and brought into the light of consciousness.

While Jerry's story fed him with continual information about the dire nature of his circumstances and the need to control everything in order to survive, Jerry's dream was actually to live in spiritual freedom. He wanted to live without having to constantly plan or think everything through; he wanted to live in an expanded state of consciousness. This kind of life was magnetically attractive to Jerry, and it also scared him to death. What if he really did get out of his head? Would he become a drooling idiot? How could he live his life if he didn't think and plan everything out ahead of time? How does one function logically and make responsible decisions about things like finances or obeying the speed limit or taking out the garbage when you're in your heart?

For Jerry, it wasn't just about remembering that he could choose his behavior and choose to come from his heart; it was also about welcoming and embracing his *fear* of doing precisely that. For a long time Jerry had been trying to surrender at exactly the same time he was resisting. The friction made him so uncomfortable he would sweat. He came to recognize that there was a space between the story and him. As he was able to put words to it and deconstruct it, he found the space to breathe into it. It was then his Ego began to relax and unwind itself altogether.

Jerry finally experienced a whole being breakthrough. This kind of transformation registers as a shift on the cellular level, leaving you living life with expanded and clarified vision. When your whole being breaks through and taps into your Heart's Wisdom, the awareness and practice of living your life from the heart has gone so deeply into your cells that it is now fully integrated. You are living from your heart, and you are connected to the Divine. This connection is bound to show in all of your actions and decisions, as the very fabric of who you are has transformed. When you enter into your Heart Wisdom you operate from a place of unity and oneness instead of a place of separation, and you feel whole. Thus you create your very own heaven on earth.

Believe it or not, this heavenly experience can happen to us anywhere, anytime.

The Gold at the "End" of My Rainbow

Along my journey, I have had some potent healing experiences. In listening to my heart wisdom, I have been guided to explore and participate in some methods of healing that are, let us say, on the road less traveled. Many of these have included Native American sweat lodges and vision quests, water fasting, colon therapy, a vast array of healing modalities from Reiki and theta healing to pranic healing and rebirthing, lubricolor quantum light healing and even crystal healing. And last, but surely not least, is shamanic healing,

Shamanic healing, more specifically Peruvian shamanism, is much more than a healing modality; it is actually a cosmology, a way of intelligent, harmonious living, and it holds a very special place in my heart. It was along this shamanic healing path that I underwent a particularly miraculous healing.

One aspect of shamanic healing involves plant spirit medicine work. The word medicine itself comes from the root word *medi*, which means middle or center. Medicine really means that which brings you back to center, or, to put it another way, that which helps restore balance or connection to one's true self. Plant spirit medicine involves working with the living intelligence of specific plants as the means to achieving this end. It is said that Indian medicine men, or "shamans," adopted the word medicine in the sense of "magical influence."

"The magic" of plant spirit medicine has been practiced in ceremonial gatherings for thousands of years by indigenous cultures, and, thanks to the books of people like Carlos Castaneda, Alberto Villoldo, Ralph Metzner and Pablo Amaringo, is now enjoying resurgence across the globe. I could write a whole book on the miraculous journeys I have had with this work, but for now, I trust that one powerful and astonishing story should suffice!

It was one recent ceremony with the plant medicine Ayahuasca that proved to be the *piece de resistance* in my long healing journey. For those of you who have never experienced or been exposed to this sacred plant, it is a traditional shamanic elixir known as the Queen of the Forest or the Mother of Life, and is administered by shamans and in prayer throughout the world. It is served like a tea in ceremony circles and each experience holds its own magic. The healing that came forth for me in this particular ceremony is what actually allowed me to complete this book. I experienced deep healing of my heart from anxiety, fear of death and profound heartbreak. The journey was the culmination of years of inner work to heal my heart. The healing occurred in a flash, but the flash was the result of years of commitment, devotion and practice in following the path of my Heart Wisdom.

On this particular majestic evening, as we began the deep dive inward into "ceremony", the medicine began to take effect very quickly. Sometimes it happens that way, and this one shot out like a rocket. The first couple of hours were an intense purification of my mind. I could see and feel my mind being cleansed and recalibrated at the speed of light. The healing power of this inner light incinerated patterns of confusion, darkness and insanity, freeing up space for something new to happen. That something new I would soon come to see as nothing short of miraculous. Because light moves beyond space and time and, therefore, is not restricted by space or time, it can connect you to the level of your soul, thereby healing some very deep stuff very quickly.

After the purification part of the process, I knew something had cleared and shifted, because I felt totally open and connected to a profound intelligence. Everything was accessible to me. It was like my mind had been upgraded from a Pentium 1 to a Pentium 12 processor. At that moment, I felt the call to step outside.

As I walked outside, my attention turned to my heart (as it usually does), and I picked up where I had left off from my last deep exploration of my heart. I became aware that my heart still felt broken from a devastating heartbreak from a relationship that ended many years prior. Since it has become such a natural process for me, I immediately engaged the Heart Wisdom practice. Soon I became aware of an intense feeling of heartbreak, and started to track the feelings back into the center of my heart.

At that very instant of extreme openness and receptivity, something extraordinary happened. Deep within my heart, where, just moments before, I had been feeling the pain of an old heartbreak, I felt a sensation that I can only describe as my heart being "energetically cauterized!" I could literally feel the emotional wound sealing up and healing over. In one moment my heart was broken, and in the next it was not. My heart had healed!

And even more astonishing, in the very next instant, I watched my mind recalibrate the experience. I actually "saw" the program of heartbreak become unprogrammed and dissolve as though it had never existed. As my being was recalibrated to its soul's intelligence, the heartbreak became deleted from the algorithm of my life!

Although the heartbreak had felt very real, I could now see that it was just a program that had been made up. My heart was never broken. What's more, I was shown that the heart can *never* be broken. On the level of soul, there is no heartbreak, because there isn't anything that is wrong or broken or needing to be fixed. As I connected on the level of soul, my heart was restored to its natural state. I felt the truth that there really is nothing wrong, ever. We just cover our hearts with our conditioned mind stuff. Once that stuff is unraveled, you can see the heart was never broken in the first place.

The mind is powerful.

In *The Matrix*, while having an experience in the simulated world, Neo injures his lip. Feeling the blood on his lip, he asks Morpheus, "How can this be real?" Morpheus then says, "Your mind makes it real."

The mind does indeed make it real. But it is not the truth. For truth only lies within your heart and soul.

On that extraordinary evening, through the power of Peruvian shamanic wisdom, I came face to face with the astonishing power of my soul... and it was in that moment that the process of Heart Wisdom, which had been gestating within my soul and my practice for so long, was finally born!

I had come full circle with the healing of my heart and connected with my heart's wisdom. My inner intelligence had revealed itself in full force. I had witnessed firsthand the power that lies within, and the magic that resides within the Wisdom of the Heart. If I hadn't experienced it myself, I wouldn't have believed it. This is the gift that I believe I came here to receive and to pass on.

I believe that we all come here for a purpose. The supreme intelligence of life doesn't make mistakes. We are not here by accident. People endlessly seek their life's purpose, and most are looking in all the wrong places. They scour their minds to discover that precious gem of purpose—to excavate the gold that lies within their soul. But the problem is that the answers they are seeking do not come within the domain of the mind, no matter how hard they look. It's like going to a bakery to buy tires! Your purpose, the gold you truly seek, is in the treasure of your very own heart!

During that miraculous healing experience, I felt connected to my soul in a way I had never felt before. It was as if for the first time I really knew who I was. That may sound like a dramatic statement, but it's the truth.

This book is about the healing of your heart, which is the gateway to your soul and your doorway to lasting peace, liberation and fulfillment. It is my hope that the practices in this book have already begun to help you unravel the tensions and stress patterns that constrict your heart's innate wisdom from flowing freely. Your heart is the hub of your feeling nature and when you begin to release the restrictions in your heart, you can connect more authentically not only with who you are but also with the people and the world around you.

Out there in the world at large we have literally lost touch with one another. We don't feel connected anymore, and as a result, we continue, albeit unconsciously, to hurt each other and to perpetuate a way of living that is detrimental to our health and the health of others and the world we live in.

When we feel disconnected from our hearts we tend to go into fear. Fear is a part of life, but being afraid is optional. You now have the power of your own Heart Wisdom to guide you, to change your life, to give you strength and clarity, to be a radiant light and a shining example for others.

Through your Heart Wisdom you now have the power to change the world. Are you ready?

HEART WISDOM KEY NUMBER NINE

Living Heart Wisdom

Now that you have gone through the Heart Wisdom process, done the exercises and visited my Web site and taken advantage of the free audios, chances are you have already started noticing many positive changes. Now here's the payoff.

Remember that exercise you did at the end of Chapter Two? Now's the time to get it out and reread everything you wrote down that you had thought you wanted or had acquired in the past six months, or were planning to acquire in the near future. Then read through all the reasons why you thought that that having that thing would make you happy. Now ask yourself:

- How many of these things do I still feel are necessary for me to feel good about myself and my life, or to know true happiness? When I think about having those things now, does it make my heart sing?

- Will having any of these things connect me any deeper to my Heart Wisdom?

- Now cross off/delete all of the things you no longer need or desire—all of the things, that object, that achievement, that whatever that you thought would give you happiness, and are now not aligned with your Heart Wisdom.

- Take out a new piece of paper or open to a clean page in your journal and make a new list: your Heart Wisdom List.

- Write down all the things that are important to you now, all the things you truly require in order to make you happy, and that serve your Heart's Wisdom and nourish your soul *now*!

Now that you have completed this exercise you may find you are surprised at the results. There may be many things that no longer have deep meaning for you that were very important the first time you did the exercise. And there may be a few you are not ready to let go of yet. Don't worry. Heart Wisdom is an ever unfolding process that takes you deeper into yourself and your heart, and brings you farther and farther into the light of love. "The force is with you."

Have a blessed journey…

Nine Ways to Stay Connected to Your Heart Wisdom

1. Live it!

2. Listen often to the free downloads of the Heart Wisdom exercises and meditations

3. Sign up for my Heart Wisdom Newsletter, receive free coaching tips and advance notice of my free Heart Wisdom Webinars: www.heartwisdom/com/newsletter

4. Stay "tuned in" with the Heart Wisdom blog: *www.heartwisdom.com/blog*

5. Support your friends, family, co-workers and everyone you care about by sharing your Heart Wisdom experience.

6. Direct people to the website *www.heartwisdom.com* to sample the first chapter as a free gift. Or simply gift them a copy of this book.

7. When you are done with this book, pay it forward by leaving it somewhere as a gift for someone else to benefit from, like in a coffee shop, library, airport, or on a train, a bus or in a friend's car…

8. Write a review. Tell the world why you love this book at *www.amazon.com, www.barnesandnoble.com, www.borders.com* or *www.goodreads.com*

9. Suggest *Heart Wisdom* to your book club, church, school, and/or spiritual group to do a reading/inspirational Talk.

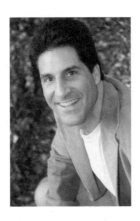

About the Author

Russell Feingold is a master healer, transformational coach and professional speaker. Born with the unique gift of being highly energetically sensitive, Russell had a mystical experience at the age of twenty that awakened him to a reality he didn't know existed: a beauty, intelligence, and love that changed the way he understood and experienced life forever. Over the last fifteen years, he has personally helped thousands of people, including many well known authors and leaders.

Russell has presented at events alongside such well-known authors and presenters as Robert F. Kennedy, Jr., Caroline Myss, Rev. Michael Bernard Beckwith (The Secret), Andrew Harvey and T. Harve Eker, and has been noted in LA Weekly's "Best of LA" for his Transformational Coaching.

His programs and 9-step Heart Wisdom process guide you on a magical journey that heals your heart from past wounds and opens you to sacred union with yourself and others.